DATE DUE

World University Library

The World University Library is an international series
of books, each of which has been specially commissioned.
The authors are leading scientists and scholars from all over
the world who, in an age of increasing specialisation, see the
need for a broad, up-to-date presentation of their subject.
The aim is to provide authoritative introductory books for
university students which will be of interest also to the general
reader. The series is published in Britain, France, Germany,
Holland, Italy, Spain, Sweden and the United States.

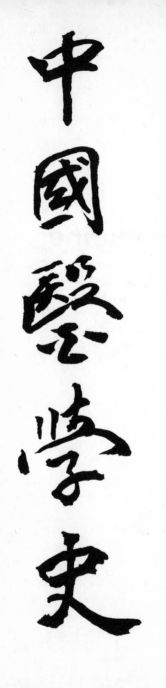

中國醫學史

Pierre Huard and
Ming Wong

Chinese Medicine

translated from the French by Bernard Fielding

World University Library

McGraw-Hill Book Company
New York Toronto

© Pierre Huard and Ming Wong 1968
Translation © George Weidenfeld and Nicolson Limited 1968
Library of Congress Catalog Card Number: 67-14680
Phototypeset by BAS Printers Limited,Wallop, Hampshire, England
Printed by Officine Grafiche Arnoldo Mondadori, Verona, Italy

Contents

Introduction

Since the end of the seventeenth century the West has created a mechanical image of the world which has been a powerful stimulus to all scientific and technical development (with the exception of the human sciences, which are considerably behind the others). It might in fact be said that a certain level of material comfort and civilisation is not equally beneficial to the different elements of culture and that some are sacrificed to it. That is not of course the case with scientific medicine, which has found a chosen place in this state of affairs. Its accelerated development has quickly set it apart from its less fortunate Eurasian and American Indian sisters.

These ancient medical systems doubtless appear to be obsolete, and the ground has to be very carefully searched in order to discover the few examples of exceptional interest, but it is an interest which is by no means negligible.

In all the developing countries we are in fact confronted with an economy at two levels, the one more or less uncontaminated and indigenous, the other already Western. China is no exception to this rule. There Western medicine has reached a very high level in certain particularly favoured urban areas. Elsewhere, for want of the necessary substructure, it has not yet been able to drive out popular medicine which, by its very definition, is admirably suited to the economic and psychological condition of the peasant masses who support it. At little expense it happily fulfils an essential social function which nothing could replace. This traditional medicine (which has its own 'officials' and healers) is of interest not only to doctors through its extremely varied therapeutics, but also to linguists, ethnologists, sociologists, psychologists and all who are aware of the fruitful possibilities of a medically informed approach to the study of China and its potentialities for modern science.

Its complexity, however great, is manifestly incapable of giving us a complete picture of the art of healing and the 'techniques of the body'. Only a comparative study, in time and space, of all known medical systems will make possible the formulation of a medicine which will then be no longer that of a specific civilisation but will deserve to be called universal. On that day, for doctors,

8

Walt Whitman's 'great rondure' of the world will indeed be an accomplished fact and a new medical humanism will have been born.

In such a perspective Chinese medicine acquires an enhanced significance. We have tried first of all to show the evolution of classical opinion and its mental context, the concepts of which, valid throughout the Far East, have no 'grip' on Western behaviour. Furthermore we have accorded a special significance to the present development of public health in mainland China, as it is to be seen in the second decade of the People's Republic.

Chinese medicine is not yet well known. Owing to the lack of technical glossaries certain classical works present difficulties of interpretation even to scholars of Chinese, and their translation into Western languages poses many problems. We are therefore grateful to all our Chinese correspondents, and particularly to the late Professor Li T'ao and Dean S. S. Wong for the information they have so kindly provided for us. We also thank our friend Dr R. A. Husson who has so freely allowed us the use of his many excellent translations.

1 The evolution of Chinese Medicine

An appreciation of the difference between the norms of Western historians and those of the Chinese chroniclers is essential to an understanding of the development of Chinese medicine.

Very early in their history the eastern Mediterranean countries acquired systems of chronology with fixed starting points allowing the calculation of years backwards and forwards. Instead of the Greek, Roman, Jewish, Christian and Islamic linear eras, China used a chronology of compartments: a series of temporal cycles shut off from each other, the largest being the dynastic periods, then the reigns of the emperors, subdivided to the end of the Yüan dynasty into periods of still smaller *nien-hao* (or 'styles of the reign'), which in their turn are cut up into years, seasons, months and days. Each historical fact is thus situated in an extremely precise framework, according to an exact chronology which gives Chinese annals a great historical value unknown in other civilisations. But this system is not without its disadvantages:

1 It leads to a very concrete conception of the duration of time as a series of moments without continuity.
2 It becomes difficult to extract a fact from the framework in which it has been so carefully set.
3 It results in compilations which are good moral or administrative guides, i.e. annals, but never in attempts at explanation which form a principal characteristic of historical writing.

Thus, on a more general plane, Chinese culture is unacquainted with the notions of evolution, comparison and context. Although there may be precise knowledge of what happened in a given period of time, there has never been any serious attempt to compare a period with those preceding and following it. This has led to a timeless atmosphere in which there is no fundamental differentiation of scientific data, works of art, or techniques separated by many centuries. There is a tendency to put on the same plane paintings which are chronologically very different and to include under the same title in the same work chapters of very dissimilar periods of origin. In medicine it will appear neither astounding nor impossible to compare the ancient *Nei-ching* ('The Classic of

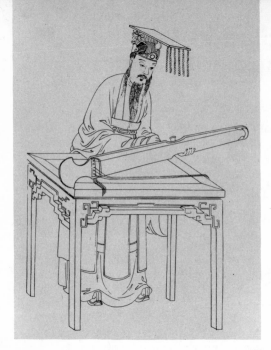

Left Shen Nung, the legendary emperor and patron of agriculture and herbal medicine. The pharmacopoeia which bears his name lists 365 drugs and is the first materia medica of China. The work was in fact compiled by an Early Han dynasty writer, whose sources go back only as far as the fourth century BC.

Right Fu Hsi, another of the 'Three August Rulers'. Traditionally the author of *The Canon of Changes*, a work of the Chou dynasty dating from the ninth to eighth century BC.

Internal Medicine') with a recent work compiled in accordance with the standards of contemporary scientific medicine; it would even be possible for the latter to be regarded as inspired by the *Nei-ching*. Whereas since Hippocrates countless classics (some of no great age) have become obsolete in the West, the *Nei-ching* still holds the prestige of antiquity and scientific interest. This is a medical attitude which cannot be disregarded, especially since it has survived all political revolutions; it gives Chinese medicine its timeless, monolithic aspect in which, however, each generation has left its mark, usually discernible on careful examination.

Early Medicine

We have almost no knowledge of the medicine of the prehistoric civilisations. Three legendary emperors are connected with this period: Fu Hsi, to whom is attributed the 'Canon of Changes' (*I-ching*), regarded as the most ancient of Chinese books, Shen Nung, the father of agriculture and herbal therapy, and Huang Ti, the creator of ritual and of medicine. Although the last-mentioned

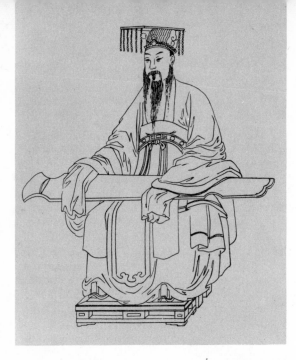

had a cenotaph (recently restored) erected in his honour by the Emperor Wu Ti (140–87 BC) of the Han dynasty at Hwangling (one hundred and fifty miles from Sian), the lives of the 'Three August Rulers' remain completely in the field of legend. Shen Nung was no more the compiler of the first *Pen-ts'ao* ('Treatise on Medicine') than was Huang Ti the compiler of the *Nei-ching*.

The earliest medical texts are to be found in the *Tso-chuan*. They cannot be considered for certain to date earlier than 540 BC.[1] This does not mean that Chinese medicine begins at that date – it is certainly of much earlier origin – but it could have been conveyed by recitation, or by texts engraved on bone of which all trace is lost today, but which may well have existed, since the medical symbols date back to the thirteenth or fourteenth centuries BC.

The period of the organisation of ritual (*Li-chi*) and administration (*Chou-li*) sees the first corporation of doctors (*Yi*) independent of priests and magicians (*Wu*). This body's first known representative was Pien Ts'io, a more or less legendary figure who probably personifies several historical characters. He is thought to have lived *c*. 430–350. He already knew the pulse rate (*mo-fa*) as a basis for diagnosis and prognosis. The authorship of the *Nan-ching* (a classic on difficult problems) has been attributed to him. From this period onwards China borrowed from India and Iran. Thus Tsou Yen (*c.*305–240 BC) introduced to the Far East the idea of the five elements (wood, earth, metal, fire, water), their mutual genesis and destruction, after which the Chinese medical system was built upon the doctrine of the elements and vital spirits like its Indian, Greek and later Arab counterparts, and was opened to the influence of the alchemists' school of thought. This occurred during the fourth and third centuries BC as the result of a reciprocal reaction between Western chemical notions (the Babylonian preparation of mercury, the Indo-European idea of the immortality of the soul) and Chinese conceptions. It very soon directed Chinese doctors towards a knowledge of poisons and of herbal and mineral remedies, dietetics, the quest for immortality drugs, respiratory techniques, physical culture and the study of sex.

Medicine in the Ancient Empire (206BC–AD580)

Chinese feudalism was to crumble in the fratricidal wars of the Contending States. The king of Ch'in (modern Shensi) obtained mastery of the other kingdoms 'by fire and the sword'. Under the name of Ch'in Shih Huang Ti (221–210 BC) 'First August Lord Ch'in' he built the Great Wall and gave the Empire its social, political and administrative structure from which scholars were excluded. Almost immediately after his death the Han dynasty (206 BC–AD 220) succeeded the Ch'in. Gradually the scholars took up their positions again and the Chinese military empire was rapidly transformed into a tradition-conscious monarchy, anxious to re-establish its connection 'beyond the centuries of the words, with the saints and sages of the golden age'.[2] After a period of splendour it was split up into the Three Kingdoms (220–280). In spite of an ephemeral restoration, effected by the Western Chin dynasty (265–316), no resistance was made against the barbarian invasions, and so there began a period of confusion comparable to the beginning of the Middle Ages in the West[3] but much shorter, during which the barbaric dynasties of the north opposed for the first time the national dynasties of the south.

Contemporary with the Roman and Sassanian empires, the Han Empire (206 BC–AD 220) represents the emergence of Chinese civilisation at world level. By the Silk Road (122 BC), the Burma Road (115 BC) and the maritime routes, China began direct or indirect contact with Iran, India, South-East Asia and the Mediterranean.

In the shadow of the *pax sinica* all forms of scientific thought were stimulated during the two centuries preceding this period and during the one following it. Medicine joined in this great intellectual movement and found expression in a number of works classified as follows in the Annals of the Han dynasty (*Han-shu*):

1 *I-ching* ('Classics of Medicine').
2 *Ching-fang* ('Collection of Prescriptions').
3 *Fang-chung* (treatises on the bedroom, or on sex and general hygiene).
4 *Shen-sien* (methods and prescriptions for immortality).

All these works are lost. Only the 'Classic of Internal Medicine', attributed in legend to the 'Yellow Emperor' Huang Ti, has reached us.

The three great masters of this period were Shun-yü Yi, Chang Chung-ching and Hua T'o.

Shun-yü Yi, a native of Lin-tzu (Shantung), was probably born *c.*215 BC.[4] At the age of twenty-eight he began to study medicine under his first master Chung-sun Chuang. He then became for three years the pupil of Ch'eng Yang-ch'ing (*c.*177 BC) who handed on to him his secret prescriptions (*pi-fang*). At this time he was put in charge of the public granaries (*ts'ang*) of Ts'i, which caused him to be given the courtesy title of 'Father Tsang' (Ts'ang Chung).

For ten years he was both doctor and civil servant. Then (167 BC) he was brought before the Imperial court of justice (on an unknown charge), condemned to corporal punishment, but pardoned. Between 164 and 154 BC he became the doctor of several princes and kings. After the defeat of his last client, Liou Tsiang-lu, Shun-yü Yi found himself in a difficult situation. From 154 onwards we have no further trace of him. It is possible that he was only able to keep his position under the threat of the purge by writing a report[5] outlining the sum of his medical experience. In this report he was made to state the ailments he was able to treat, the names of his masters, his patients and books as well as his diagnoses and the treatments he was then prescribing. Briefly summarised his replies are:

(*i*) Twenty-five observations compiled to a very logical scheme (anamnesis, clinical examination, diagnosis, prognosis, treatment, pathogenesis, discussion of the symptoms and explanation of the treatment). Among them can be recognised: cirrhosis of the liver, strangulated hernia, traumatic lumbago, a peritoneal abscess, infantile quinsy, a paludal (?) abscess, pyelo-nephritis, congestion of the lungs, an attack of gout, helminthiasis, an undefined abdominal syndrome, an intrathoracic pulmonary or pleural abscess, creeping paralysis, retention of the urine and haemoptysis.

(*ii*) A library consisting of works which have all disappeared except for the *Nei-ching*. Despite Shun's respect for the writers of antiquity he considered that their advice was to be followed only when it was not contradictory to facts, for it is impossible to introduce the complexity of clinical instruction into a rigid system. The formalism of China can thus be said to have worked against Shun-yü Yi's effective influence.

Chang Chung-ching, the Chinese Hippocrates, was the codifier of Chinese symptomatology and therapeutics. He was the first to differentiate clearly between '*yang*' and '*yin*' symptoms. A native of Nie-Yang (today the administrative district of Nanyang in the province of Honan), he was born *c*. 158–166.[6] Under the reign of the Emperor Ling Ti (168–188) of the later Han dynasty Chang Chung-ching was given the title '*Hiao-lien*' (graduate of the second degree), and during the period of Kien-an (196–219) he became '*T'ai-shou*' (administrative officer) of Changsha. He acquired a reputation as an encyclopedist and learnt medicine from Chang

Pai-tsu, also a native of Nie-Yang. Chang Chung-ching compiled an authoritative work entitled *Shang-han lun* (treatise on ailments caused by cold), or *Treatise on Fevers*, often translated in error as *Treatise on Typhoid* (*Shang-han* being the modern term for typhoid). It was subsequently divided into *Shang-han lun* proper and *Chin-kwei yao-lio fang* (summary dealing with the prescriptions of the Golden Box). It is as significant a work as the *Nei-ching*.

The *Shang-han tsa-ping lun* (treatise in sixteen chapters on various ailments caused by the cold) is still the bedside book of the traditional young practitioner. The most esteemed classical edition is one consisting of wood-engravings by Ch'ao Ch'ai-mei of the Ming period (1368–1644) with notes by Ch'eng Wu-chi of the Sung period (about the eleventh century).[7]

Hua T'o (writing under the name of Yüan Hua) was the great surgeon of this period. He was born in the administrative district of Po in the province of Anhwei and there is some doubt as to his dates. In all probability he was born during the reign of the Emperor Shun (Yung-ho period, AD 136–41) and died during the reign of Hien Ti (thirteenth year of the Chien-an period) in 208.

His most important discoveries were in the field of anaesthetics (*ma-tsuei-fa*) and the art of abdominal section (*ch'ai-fu-shu*). He is credited with extraordinary operations of the same style as those attributed to Pien Ts'io (laparotomies, thoracotomies, grafting of organs, intestinal resections, rhinoplasties, lithotomies) carried out under general anaesthetic by Indian hemp, but difficult to accept owing to the lack of adequate instrumental equipment. The only operation we can reasonably attribute to him is the trepanation he is said to have recommended to the Emperor Ts'ao Ts'ao. But we cannot be certain, as we shall see later, whether this operation was anything more than treatment by acupuncture. Whatever the case we find here an operation known since the end of the Palaeolithic period, taking the form later of a kill-or-cure remedy for certain types of blindness, in Greece (Hippocrates) and in India, where Jivaka, who later became Buddha's doctor, used it successfully on three occasions. It is probably therefore the Chinese

16

version of an Indian operation propagated by Buddhism. But whereas China has borrowed from India numerous philosophical, linguistic, astronomical, mathematical, dialectic and therapeutic ideas, she appears to owe little to her in the field of surgery and the development of surgical instruments, in which the Indians have shown themselves superior to all the ancient peoples.

Ts'ao Ts'ao, who reigned over northern China, was suffering from violent headaches, and Hua T'o, who was consulted, probably cured him by one single operation of acupuncture. From then on Ts'ao Ts'ao tried to keep the eminent surgeon in his service, but Hua T'o escaped from the authoritarian monarch at the first opportunity. Ts'ao Ts'ao had him imprisoned and then assassinated in 208. According to legend Hua T'o tried to entrust his writings for the relief of human ills to his gaoler who was too frightened of punishment to take them. In despair Hua T'o burnt his manuscript. That is why the texts bearing his name are late, apocryphal compilations. The *Hua-shih chung-tsang ching* was in fact compiled by Sun Sing-yen (1753–1818), a bibliophile and calligrapher. His book consists of three chapters:

Chapter 1 (twenty-nine sections): the *yin-yang* duality, cold and heat, deficiency and excess, symptomatology of organs and viscera (*tsang-fu*).

Chapter 2 (twenty sections): rheumatism, anthrax, ulcers, abscesses and fatal illnesses. Diagnosis by sound and colour.

Chapter 3 (supplement): therapeutics and pharmacological prescriptions.

It is known that we owe the practice of hydrotherapy and medicinal baths to Hua T'o. The forty-nine sections of the first three chapters were the object of careful revision by Sun Sing-yen. He checked the references of the great historian Cheng Ts'iao (1104–62), who composed the *T'ung Chih*. The eight bibliographical chapters of this book are entitled *I-wen-lio* (account of artistic and literary works divided into twelve categories). The tenth category (*I-fang-lei*) deals with medicine. Sun also consulted the *Chih-chai-shu-lu*, a catalogue by Ch'en Chen-sun, a contemporary of Cheng

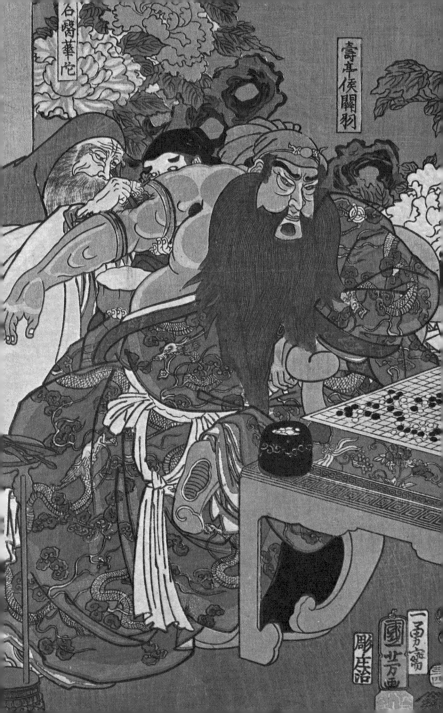

白醫華佗

壽亭侯關羽

一勇齋
國芳画

彫庄治

Ts'iao. Under the Northern Sung dynasty (960–1126) two kinds of woodcut were in existence for the printing of the *Treatise on Internal Medicine* by Hua T'o. Wu Mien-hiue, an editor of medical works of the Ming period (1368–1644) incorporated them in his collection entitled *Chu-chin i-tung cheng-mo ch'iuan-shu* ('Comprehensive Collection on the Study of the Pulse').

Hua T'o was a practitioner in acupuncture, an anatomist and a therapeutist.

When he acknowledged that acupuncture had to be used he would apply it in two or three places; he carried out the same procedure in the case of moxa if it was indicated by the nature of the affection to be treated. But, if the source of the ailment was in those parts of the body where the needle, the moxa or liquid applications could have no effect, for example in the bones, the bone marrow, the stomach or the intestines, he gave a preparation of hemp (*ma-yo*) to the patient, who, after a few moments would become as insensate as if he were completely intoxicated or deprived of life. Then he would cut open, make incisions or amputate as required and remove the cause of the illness; but he would stitch together the tissues and apply liniments. After a certain number of days (at the end of one month according to the reckoning of the later Han period) the patient would be well again without having felt the slightest pain during the operation.

Hua T'o is thought to have published, under the title *Nei-chao-t'u*, anatomical charts showing the inside of the human body. They have come down to us and enjoy a great reputation. As a therapeutist he used the first anaesthetics, *ma-fei-san* (Indian hemp), sutures, antiseptics, ointments to cure inflammations, anthelmintics for ascarides (*huei*) notably *ta-suan* (*Allium scorodoprasum* L.), with an admixture of vinegar.

The biography of Hua T'o is related in the historical novel of the Three Kingdoms, (*San Kuo Chih Yen I*) in connection with the wound of General Kuan Yun Chang, who received a poisoned arrow in his right arm. Hua T'o operated by cutting down to the bone and applying an ointment. It is reported that the patient was able to move his arm as soon as the wound had been stitched. This episode is a classic and has inspired many texts and engravings.

In the Kiangsu province, at Siuchou, a stele honouring his memory is still preserved. In the Po district of Anhwei the 'birthplace of Hua' and the 'temple of the ancestor Hua' are still to be found. Thus for nearly seventeen hundred years tradition has kept alive the veneration of this master of medicine.

His reputation in the history of obstetrics is equally famous. He diagnosed the intra-uterine death of a twin caused by the haemorrhage consequent upon the birth of the first child. As the obstetrician had not taken the necessary precautions, Hua T'o relieved the mother by acupuncture before delivering the still-born child whose body was already black. He was interested in the study of drugs and trained the famous pharmacologist Wu P'u. He noticed that physical culture facilitated the digestion and circulation and strengthened the body. He also invented the *wu-chin-hi*, the game of the five animals (the tiger, the stag, the bear, the monkey and the crane). The *niao-hi* (the bird game) facilitates breathing. The arms are spread out as the bird raises its wings. The monkey game (*yuan-hi*) teaches the art of climbing, and so forth. Wu P'u lived for more than ninety years by practising these methods.

Other eminent medical men of the Han period are Huang-Fu Mi (215–82), the author of the classic on acupuncture, and Wang Shu-ho (265–317), whose pulse classic, translated into Tibetan, Arabic and Persian during the Middle Ages, was to influence students of the pulse via Western translations as late as the seventeenth and eighteenth centuries. It was under the Han dynasty that the classical doctrine of medicine was formulated.

We now arrive at the great period of Taoism which stretches from the third century BC to the seventh century AD.

Ko Hung (281–340), one of the greatest Tao alchemists and pathologists, born at Kiuyung (Tanyang, Kiangsu), had a difficult youth. He worked as a wood-cutter in order to buy writing materials. Having little inclination for pleasure, he readily gave himself up to reading the works of antiquity and practised breathing exercises. He became one of the best disciples of his uncle Ko Hiuan who taught him to search for the elixir of life. At the time

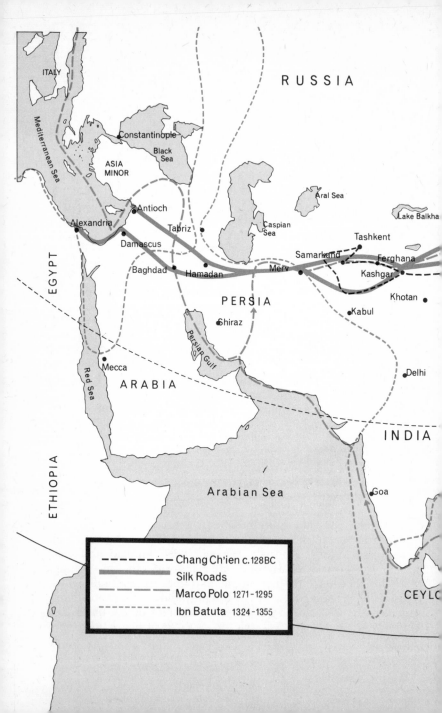

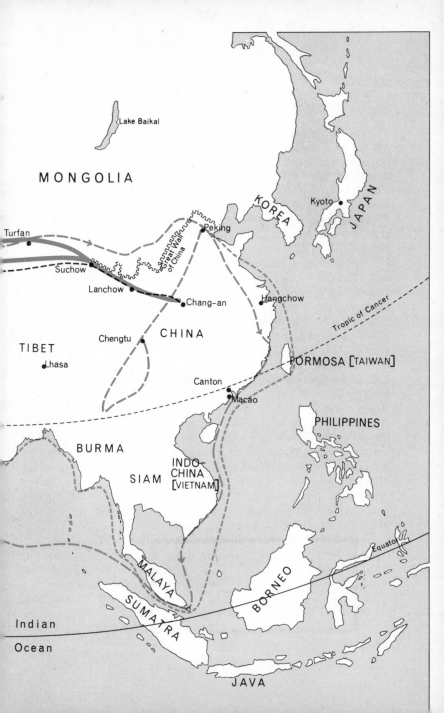

of Shih Ping's revolt during the T'ai-an period (302–3) Ko Hung
was given a captaincy and put down the rebellion. Promoted to
the post of military adviser to the Governor of Canton, he became
a man of the south and refused all honours and offers from the
Court. Hearing of the cinnabar of Chiao-chih (Annam) he was
anxious to visit that area and asked for a position there, which the
Emperor granted him although he considered it too modest for the
great scholar. But his friend the Governor kept him back, and Ko
Hung finally stayed in the Lo Fu Mountains in order to seek the
elixir of life and develop the *Tao*. He died at the age of eighty-one,
and according to legend his body after death gave the feeling of
incredible lightness, as though the clothing had been emptied of
the body; Ko Hung had become a 'divine immortal'.

Ko Hung wrote under the name of Pao-p'u Tzu. He composed
a treatise on alchemy, dietetics and magic, the *Pao-p'u Tzu nei-wai-
p'ien* (*c.* 326), the most remarkable work of modern Taoism, and
two important medical works: 'The Medications of the Golden
Box' (*Chin-kuei-yo-fang*), and first-aid measures (*Chou-hou pei-tsi
fang*) completed later by T'ao the Hermit's book of a *Hundred
Recipes*. He had a very clear idea of preventive medicine. In the
chapter *Yang-shen* of the *Pao-p'u Tzu nei-wai-p'ien* there is a list of
the methods of prolonging life and avoiding illness: put on clothes
before feeling cold, eat before feeling hungry, do not eat to capacity,
take care over the eating of raw food, avoid draughts after drinking
alcohol, do not stay awake or sleep too long, do not sleep in the
open air or with shoulders uncovered. He advises work without
over-exertion, eating in moderation especially before sleep, rising
at cock-crow and ending activity at sunset.

He further formulated two rules of longevity: *Tao-Yin:* strengthen
the *ch'i* (breath) by respiratory methods aiming to 'reject the old
(*ch'i*) in order to receive the new (*ch'i*)'. *Fu-she:* augment the
blood supply (*hiue*) by the consumption of foods and drugs.

His respiratory technique was expounded as follows: man is in
the air as air (the *ch'i*, breath) is in man. Of all the beings in the
universe there is none which can live without air. He who has

mastery over the breath caters for the internal well-being of the body (*yang-shen*). That is why he is protected from pernicious influences externally. The natural circulation of the breath follows a rule: from midnight to midday is the period of dead breath (*szu-ch'i*). Living air must be frequently inhaled. Breath technique (*yin-ch'i*: the intake of breath through the nose) is to inhale a large amount and to exhale little. The breathing is held, then stopped. Exhalation is slow and silent. When this exercise has been fully mastered the breath can be held until one has counted up to a thousand. This is called *t'ai-si* (rudimentary breathing).

In pathology Ko Hung is to be credited with the first description of smallpox (five centuries before the Arabian Rhazes, 864–925), which was brought into China by the Huns. As the new year approached, we are told, there was a seasonal affection in which pustules appeared on the face and spread rapidly all over the body. They looked like burns covered with white starch and re-formed as soon as they were broken. The majority of those affected died if they were not immediately treated. After recovery purplish black scars remained. The epidemic disappeared at the end of the season. It was in the fourth year of Yung Huei; a malignant miasma had travelled from the west to the east with some prisoners, hence the name *lu-ch'uang* for the disease. (*Chou-hou pei-tsi fang*, chapter 2). Measles had earlier been isolated by Chih Fa-tsun, *c*.307.

Ko Hung described phthisis thus:

the *shih-chu* or *kuei-chu* generally gives rise to a high fever, sweating, asthenia, unlocalised pains making all positions difficult and slowly bringing about consumption and death, after which the disease is transferred to the relations until the whole family has been wiped out. (*Chou-hou pei-tsi fang*, chapter 1.)

He recorded that

beriberi (*chio-ch'i*), appearing south of the mountains, has reached the area east of the Blue River. It is not progressive. Occasionally the patient feels indeterminate pains, swelling in the legs, a sudden weakness on rising, paraesthesis of the lower abdomen, sometimes excessive heat or cold. Unless treated early the disease reaches the abdomen and the patient dies. (*Chou-hou pei-tsi fang*, chapter 3.)

Silk-worm of the *Ailantus* (*ch'u-chi*) or *Attacus Cynthia* Drury (1773). A lepidopteran with grey elytra and red wings known by the name 'Red lady' (*hung-niang-tzu*). Effective against perverse breaths of the heart and abdomen, and against impotence. From Liou Wen-t'ai's *pen-ts'ao*.

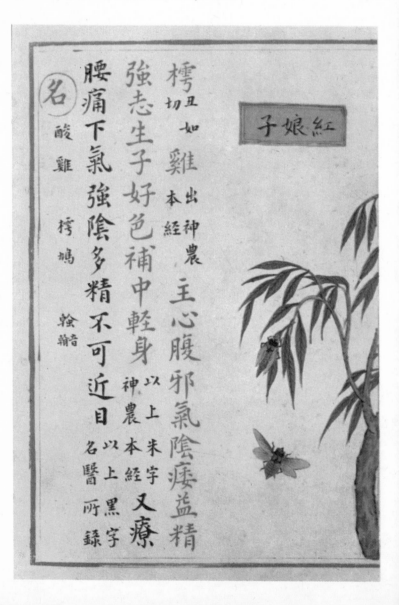

樗雞出神農　本經　主心腹邪氣陰痿益精

強志生子好色補中輕身　以上朱字　神農本經　又療

腰痛下氣強陰多精不可近目　名醫所錄

丑如雞　樗切

名　酸雞　樗鳩　乾音

The tiger (*hu*), from the
Pen-ts'ao p'in-huei tsing-yao composed
c. 1505 by Liou Wen-t'ai. Tiger
bones are effective against perverse
breaths, fears and palpitations. Tiger
balm and wine are still in use today.

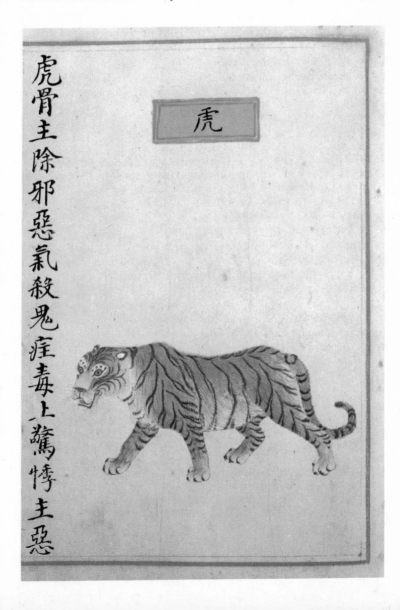

虎骨主除邪惡氣殺鬼疰毒止驚悸主惡

虎

In 'prisoners' jaundice' (thus implying its contagiousness) Ko Hung described hepatitis, its incubation period and the development of its effect on the urine.

This disease begins with a lassitude in the limbs, then the eyes go yellow and the colour progressively covers the whole body. The urine gives white paper the colour of the sap of young shoots.
(*Chou-hou pei-tsi fang*, chapter 2.)

Bubonic plague

is a disease of malignant nodules (*ngo-mo-ping*) which suddenly appear in the flesh, the size of a peach or a pear, the smallest being the size of a bean. They spread over the body in both directions, there is a high fever, fistulous adenopathy and shivering. Of frequent occurrence in the south, this disease is brutal in its early stages, it is toxic and is fatal if it gets into the abdomen. (*Chou-hou pei-tsi fang*, chapter 6.)

He described acute lymphangitis

as 'a network of red veins, resembling earth-worms, breaking out on the skin'. (Chapter 6.)

He noted the long incubation period for rabies. He wrote of glanders:

If a man with a wound mounts a sweating horse, either through a hair entering the wound, or simply through contact with the animal's breath, a painful swelling develops and is fatal if it enters the abdomen. (*Chou-hou pei-tsi fang*, chapter 7.)

Ko Hung's notes on internal medicine described a curious parasitic disease:

Sand-lice live in the earth and in water. They attack those who walk through grass at dawn and at dusk after rain has fallen, or those who bathe. They are rarely to be found in vegetation dried by the sun. No bigger than the tip of a hair, they can be seen in the skin like the frond of an ear of corn, very painful at the slightest disturbance. At first they can be extracted with a needle, and if they are put on the finger-nail they are mobile and red in colour like cinnabar. In the early stages of the disease something like a small seed which causes a sharp pain can be seen or felt under the skin. Three days later the joints are stiff and painful, an intermittent fever occurs, the reddened skin ulcerates; if the insect is not extracted it penetrates down to the bones, causing death. (*Chou-hou pei-tsi fang*, chapter 7.)

Kuang Ho-ling (1959) explains this pyrexia as a fever caused by *Trombiculidae*. The *Pao-p'u Tzu nei-wai-p'ien* insisted on hypaesthesia and cutaneous numbness as an essential sign of leprosy.

In therapeutics Ko Hung wanted to put cheap, easily found remedies within the reach of everyone. This is the object of the eight chapters of the *Chou-hou pei-tsi fang*, which bear the significant title 'prescriptions ready to hand'. The *Nei-p'ien chih-li* states:

> When I tell the common people that *li chung* pills and *sih shun* broth can cure cholera, coltsfoot and aster can cure a persistent cough, cirtomium is good for worms, angelica and peony for colic and so on . . . they doubt it or deny it and prefer to believe in wizardry.

Some of his work was the collation of old theories on the treatment of epidemic jaundice by mugwort, rhubarb and gardenia; asthma by *Ephedra vulgaris*, cinnamon, liquorice and apricot kernels; ascites by *Draba*, spurge and daphne; malaria by *Dichroa febrifuga*; dysentery and eye affections by *Coptis chinensis* Franch, etc. But as well as this, he recorded his own experiences of the use of henbane in dementia, the prohibition of salt in ascites, painting with sulphur and garlic for the prevention of tick-bites, hot-water bottles on the abdomen for gastro-enteritis.

He also gave a recipe for immortality pills based on gold, mercury, jade, sulphur, cinnabar and yellow arsenic, dissolved or mixed in herbal preparations. He was thus to contribute to the development of a mineral *materia medica* and to the discovery of the chemistry of mercury and lead, but also to the encumbering of therapeutics by immortality drugs which marks the great Taoist period.

T'ao Hung-ching (452–536) was a master Taoist who had been influenced by Buddhism. He is sometimes called the Leonardo da Vinci of China and he was indeed a mathematician and astronomer of repute, a calligrapher, and in addition studied alchemy, pharmacology and medicine.

Born at Tanyang (near Chinchiang on the Yangtze), Tao

Two acupuncture charts of
the Ming period, showing
vessels of the kidneys,
spleen and lungs.

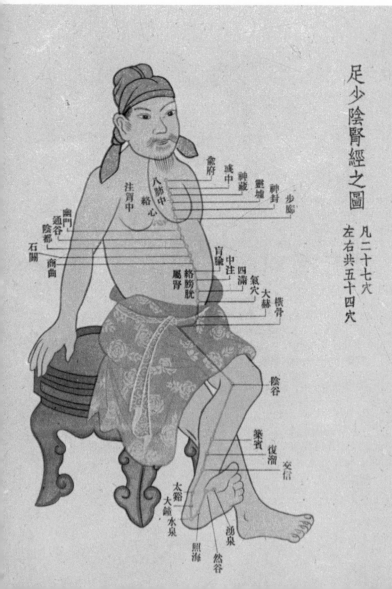

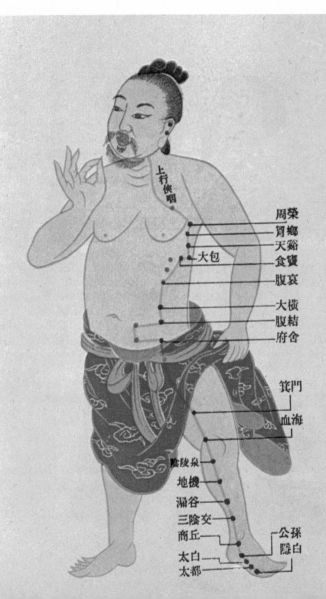

上行俠咽

周榮
胷鄉
天谿
大包
食竇
腹哀

大橫
腹結
府舍

箕門
血海

陰陵泉
地機
漏谷
三陰交
商丘
太白
太都

公孫
隱白

足太陰脾經之圖　凡二十穴　左右共四十穴

Hung-ching revealed exceptional gifts from an early age and devoted himself to study day and night. He consulted all kinds of books and particularly the *Biography of the Divine Immortals* by Ko Hung. He came to the notice of Kao Ti (479–82) of the Ts'i dynasty and became tutor to the Imperial Princes, and later Minister, but he preferred the life of a hermit and in the tenth year of the Yung Ming era he asked the Emperor for permission to withdraw to the Mao mountains. The Emperor granted him this favour and gave him five pounds of *fu-ling* and two pints of white honey so that he could continue his dietetic research. T'ao built himself a three-storeyed straw hut in which he is said to have set up a planetarium as well as pursuing his therapeutic research.

An official pharmacopoeia was in fact in existence, the *Shen-nung pen-ts'ao ching*, the ancestor of all later *Pen-ts'ao*, attributed to the legendary emperor Shen Nung. The original text of the *Pen-t'sao ching* was lost and is known to us only through an annotated edition by T'ao Hung-ching, the *Ming-i-pie-lu*, written in black ink as a setting for Shen Nung's text in red. This edition has likewise disappeared except for the introduction, which was discovered towards the end of the Ming dynasty in the famous caves of Tunhuang.

The *Pen-ts'ao ching* or *Pen-ching* compiled by T'ao contains some very old material but was composed for the greater part under the Early Han dynasty (206 BC–AD 9) by an unknown author who took the cover of a legendary name and used early sources but did not go beyond the fourth century BC.

This work deals with 365 mineral, herbal or animal drugs.[8]

Classical Medicine

After the second partition of the Early Empire, a third reunification of Chinese territory took place under the dynasties of the Middle Empire, the Sui (581–618) and the T'ang (618–906).

For the first time in the world the selection of civil servants was systematically effected by written competitive examination. There thus arose an intelligentsia formed by the *Shih* (scholar-administrators) which dissociated political power (represented by the autocracy and the plutocracy) from literary prestige and intellectual standing. This non-hereditary, fluid class formed for itself a scale of values which were very different from those of the merchants and landowners. It brought techniques of great precision into the legal administration and the supervision of the people. From the eighth century onwards contracts of sale and loan show that the finger-prints of the contracting parties have been affixed to the deed. Every foreigner entering China had to have with him a certificate bearing details of his identity and his finger-prints. The present widespread use of finger-prints for identification purposes is the result of work on early theories of the Far East carried out by Europeans living in Asia (Sir William Herschel, research from 1858 to 1871, and Henry Faulds, 1880).

From 618 to 741 the relative stability of the political situation allowed rapid development of the Chinese economy and, as a natural consequence, splendid achievements in the field of medicine. It was the golden age of the T'ang period. Unfortunately from 742 to 820 corruption, the recurrence of civil war and, from 821, the ascendancy of eunuchs in Court circles were to be expressed in a decline in the economy and an abatement of medical research. The zenith of Chinese medicine was therefore between the seventh and eighth centuries.

Medicine was reorganised, and study was approved by examinations under the control of the *T'ai-i-shu* (Grand Medical Service), formed in 624. It is one of the earliest known examples of the teaching of medicine under state supervision. Sino-Indian, Sino-Iranian, Sino-Arab and Sino-Byzantine relations were at their most prosperous. Medicine was officially controlled and important works dealt with the study of leprosy, smallpox, measles, scabies, acute and chronic dysentery, cholera, dropsy, helminthiasis, deficiency diseases (beriberi, hemeralopia, rickets, goitre) and venereal disease. Several forms of pulmonary tuberculosis were described. The pulmonary form with haemoptysis, considered contagious by Hua

Two postage stamps recently issued in China to commemorate great doctors. *Left* Sun Szu-miao (581–682), who renounced the Court for a hermit's life and in his many writings synthesised Buddhist and Chinese medical doctrines. *Right* Shen Kua (1031–95), famous in fields as diverse as architecture, agronomy, history and medicine. He formed a theory that the apparent course of the sun round the earth was not circular but elliptical.

T'o, was attributed by Sun Szu-miao to a minute creature (*ch'ung*) which ate into the lung. The same author was acquainted with the abdominal adiposity and the cervical adenopathy already described by Ko Hung. Wang T'ao contrasted the evening fever with the physical well-being of the morning, observing nocturnal perspiration and the brightness of the face 'as though painted'. Su You invented the term *ch'uan-shih* (passing on-to the corpse) to illustrate the fatal development of the disease. Ts'uei Chih-t'i treated tuberculosis of the bone by moxibustion.

Works on ophthalmology, obstetrics, surgery, acupuncture, paediatrics and *materia medica* were all in existence. Ch'ao Yuan-fang's book on etiology and symptomatology (*Chou-ping yuan-hou lun*, c. 610) is the oldest Chinese work in this category. It contains the first reference to the itch-mite in medical literature. Diabetes (already studied by Chang Chung-ching) was still confused with other ailments, as is shown by the enumeration of its symptoms: polyphagia, polydipsia, polyuria, pollakiuria, clouded urine, urine containing sugar, frigidity, edema of the lower limbs. The *Chu-chin Lu-yen* (c. 600) tries to group them in three syndromes; yet chyluria itself is defined: 'the urine is white like bean sap, it is thick and cloudy . . .'. The connection between the two was established by the *Wai-t'ai pi-yao* ('Medical Secrets of a Civil Servant'): the white urine is preceded by swelling of the feet.

On the subject of tumours, Sun Szu-miao differentiated bone tumours, adipose tumours, tumours 'of stone', tumours of the muscles, purulent tumours (ulcers) and vascular tumours.

Ch'ao Yuan-fang divided tumours into two groups: *cheng* and *chia*. The former corresponded to a permanent, palpable tumour and the latter to an incidental, modifiable or reabsorbable tumour. For him these expressions were the equivalent of *tsiu* (inflammatory tumour). The fifty-sixth 'difficulty' of the *Nan-ching* specified names according to localisation: *fei-ch'i*, of the liver; *fu-liang*, of the heart; *pi-ch'i*, of the spleen; *si-pen*, of the lung; *pen-t'un*, of the kidney. Later there was reference to a lymphangitis of secondary development: when, very hot with physical exertion,

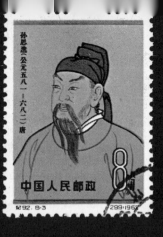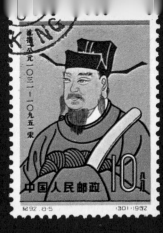

one is exposed to a cold wind. Driven back by the cold dampness, the heat withdraws into the flesh, tendons and ducts, where it forms knots. The illness takes the form of 'plaited' ropes in which there is an acute burning pain. In the leg it usually stretches from the groin to the ankle; in the arm, from below the arm-pit to the hand.

Liou Fang (1150) alluded in his new book on pediatrics (*You-you sin-shu*) to the scaly bodies which appear in certain skin diseases (*lai*). According to Li T'ao and T'ang Yu-lin (1958) the disease was pellagra.

Surgical therapy was familiar with the removal of cataract, the orthopaedic treatment of fractures and the extraction of bone sequestra. Dental caries was treated by stopping and filling with a mercurial amalgam.

'Silver paste' is listed in Su Kung's *Materia Medica* (659). Later it was also mentioned in the *Ta-kuan pen-ts'ao* by T'ang Shen-wei (*c.*1108), while during the Ming period, Liou Wen-t'ai (*Basic Materia Medica*, *c.*1505) and Li Shih-chen (1590) studied it and gave its ingredients: one hundred parts of mercury to forty-five parts of silver and nine hundred parts of tin. By trituration this gave a paste mixture which would eventually become as solid as silver. This technique, known in China for some thirteen hundred years, did not become common in Europe before Regnart (1818) and Taveau (1837).

Medical therapy was the subject of works, some of them illustrated, drawn up by an Imperial Commission. These mentioned Byzantine theriac, calomel (used for the first time in the treatment of venereal disease), *Ephedra vulgaris* for respiratory ailments, croton oil as a purgative, the dietetic treatment of deficiency diseases, in particular beriberi, of which the dry and humid forms are clearly distinguished. A high ethical code surrounded certain great doctors (like Sun Szu-miao) with the halo of the Good Samaritan.

Buddhism and Taoism were two rival powers. The Emperor T'ai Tsung the Great (600–49) was called Li Shih-min before he became emperor. As the patronymic Li belonged both to the Imperial family and to Lao Tzu (whose name was Li Erh), Lao Tzu became the ancestor of the dynasty. Taoism profited widely from this coincidence and its hermits enjoyed a high regard. A famous dispute brought Li Jung, a Taoist monk from Szechuan, and I-pao, a Buddhist monk, face to face before the Emperor Kao-tsung at Ch'ang-ngan (658). Liou Tsin-hi is thought to have written in the seventh century a *Pen-tsi ching* (book of original terms), discovered at Tunhuang, in which he denounced ignorance and cupidity as the fundamental causes of physical illness and mental suffering. In spite of their differences, Taoism and Buddhism are not incompatible. They have several points in common, one being the importance of ascesis. Ascesis is a product of the ancient Irano–Indian cultural heritage. A moral man is a healthy man whose body is pure (Zoroaster). He knows that in order to reach knowledge or ecstasy he must scorn the pleasures of the senses, avoiding their repression but working, on the contrary, towards their sublimation. He must practise prolonged meditation, accompanied by breathing exercises or in positions of complete immobility. The Indo–Iranian mentality has always remained faithful to the belief that man contains within him the power to save himself and that his own means provide him with access to the divine nature.

He who loses himself discovers himself. He who sacrifices himself wins the true life. Through the rite properly fulfilled man can redeem himself in the eyes of the gods and can save himself. Indeed he is able to rise to the divine nature and become one with it.

Thus there was formed a mental technique which radiated throughout Eurasia bearing a common characteristic: asceticism or monasticism with their great philosophies and great pantheistic or monotheistic religions: Brahminism, Buddhism, stoicism, neo-Platonism, Manichaeism, sufism, Islam, Christianity.

Sun Szu-miao (581–682) is outstanding among the monk-doctors. He was born at Huayuan (Shensi Province), the son of a scholar. From the age of seven he was a devoted and diligent student. As a youth he studied the great Taoist writers such as Lao Tzu and Chuang Tzu (fourth century BC) together with the Buddhist Canon. Early in his life he withdrew to the Tapo mountains to live as a hermit, but his renown was such that two emperors, Emperor Wen (581–604) of the Sui dynasty and Emperor Kao Tsung of the T'ang dynasty (in 660) summoned him to their courts with offers of high positions. He refused on the pretext of illness and returned to his hermitage in accordance with the tradition of the great Chinese sages. He died at an advanced age in 682 and was canonised after his death under the name of Sun Chen-jen (Sun the Wise).

The list of his principal works is as follows:

1 *Ts'ien-chin fang* ('The Thousand Costly Recipes') in thirty chapters, printed (*c.* 1068–78) by Lin Yi and republished in 1307, 1544 and 1604 by K'iao Shih-ning.[9] These editions also include the *Ts'ien-chin i* ('Supplement to the Thousand Costly Recipes').
2 *Fu-lu lun* ('Treatise on Happiness') in three chapters.
3 *Shih-sheng chen-lu* ('Articles on Hygiene'), one chapter.
4 *Shen-chung su-shu huei* (book dealing with questions 'In the Depth of the Pillow'), a study of sex, one chapter.
5 *Yin-hai ts'ing-wei* ('Exhaustive Study of the Silver Sea'), work on ophthalmology republished in 1956.
6 *San-kiao lun* ('Treatise on the Three Religions'), one chapter.

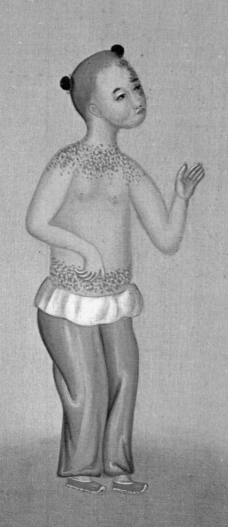

Cutaneous eruptions in children.
These pictures are from an
unpublished album in the
Bibliothèque Nationale, Paris.

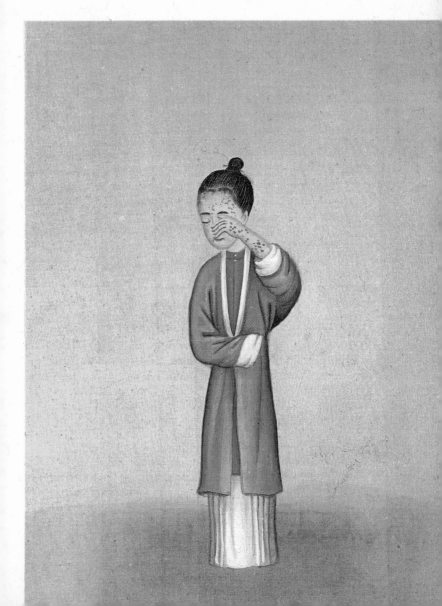

Sun Szu-miao's medical system is a compromise between the Indian doctrine of the four elements and the Chinese doctrine of five viscera. The human body is a combination of Earth, Water, Fire and Wind. When the Fire's breath is disturbed the body becomes burning-hot, if it is the breath of the Wind the pores are blocked, if it is the Water the body swells and the breathing is deep, panting and thick. If it is the breath of the Earth the four limbs are sluggish. If the Fire is suppressed the body grows cold. If the Wind stops the breathing is interrupted. If the Water fails there is no more blood. If the Earth is scattered the body bursts. If the four breaths combine their qualities the four spirits are in peaceful harmony; but should one of the breaths be disturbed, a hundred and one ailments are produced, and if the four spirits are shaken, four hundred and four ailments are produced at the same time. If eighty-one ailments are allotted to each of the viscera the result is 405 (five times eighty-one), a figure very close to that arrived at by the 101 ailments attributed to each of the four elements: $4 \times 101 = 404$.

It must not be forgotten that the authors of the periods of the Contending States (fifth to third centuries BC) and the Han dynasty (206 BC–AD 220) wrote a great deal about earlier times, but they constantly projected their own ideas on to those of the early writers, sheltering behind their names and their attainments in order to ensure a better acceptance of their own ideas and techniques.[10]

This tendency was further accentuated during the T'ang period, which is the neo-classical period *par excellence*. The most famous work is the *Nei-ching* ('The Canon of Chinese Medicine'). Its earliest fragments date back as far as three to five centuries BC, a time when it was a homogeneous composition. It appears to have been divided into two during the Ch'in period (221–206 BC).

The *Nei-ching* (eighteen chapters) is comprised of the *Su-wen* ('Simple Questions') between the Emperor Huang Ti and his ministerial advisers (principally Ki Po, nine chapters) and the *Ling-shu*, also called the *Chen-ching* (acupuncture classic in nine chapters). The *Su-wen* is in the main theoretical; the *Ling-shu* on the other hand restricts itself to practical medicine. Modifications may have taken place at the beginning of our own period. Bridgman has shown that all the passages alluding to the six receptacles (*fu*) are later than the first centuries of the Christian era. In the sixth century, under the Sui dynasty, the *Su-wen* had only eight scrolls. Under the T'ang dynasty two scrolls, the ninth and the seventh, were lost. This was the time of the classic by Wang Ping (the 'Master who reveals the Mysteries'), a doctor in the Imperial retinue who lived to be over eighty years old. He made use of many medical works: *Yuan-chu* (ten chapters), *Chao-ming yin-chih* (three chapters), etc., and practised his art during the Pao Ying period (*c.*762). His work was completed under the Sung dynasty by Lin I, Sun Chi and Sun Shao, and carried on under the Ming dynasty by Wu Mien-hiue. At least forty-nine editions were produced before the last-mentioned writer, and today three are unknown and twenty-five lost.[11]

Wang Ping appears to have used an ancient and voluminous work, now lost, in order to complete the defective text. He completely confused the chapter sequence which had already been considerably disturbed, and he filled the lacunae with extracts from other classics, adding many characters and passages of his own invention (Bridgman). It is wrong to consider the corpus of opinions expounded by him as archaic. It was formulated by successive contributions and fashioned through prolonged efforts of abstract reasoning. Fundamentals of metaphysical thought are expounded in a completely theoretical manner. These texts which so many historians of Chinese medicine have regarded as very ancient must, after analysis, be considered as composite works constantly modified from the first centuries BC to the Sui and T'ang periods.

The adaptation of these chronologically disparate texts has brought about repetitions, uncertainties, contradictions even, which a full commentary cannot always manage to clarify or reconcile. The language is, moreover, archaic, and the dialogues are composed in a rhythmic prose which has been partially trans-

The distillation of remedial wine
(from Breton's *La Chine en miniature*).

lated into English (Ilza Veith, 1949) and French (Chamfrault and Ung Kan-sam, 1957).[12]

The exposition of the *Nei-ching* text ought, as Bridgman has suggested, to be applied to all the classics. By means of an inventory of the data known at each period it would be possible to determine the share of each medical school, from the precursors with their remarkable originality down to the compilers of the Middle Empire. By such criteria Li T'ao showed that part of Sun Szu-miao's work was apocryphal and could not have been composed before the Yüan period.

After the fall of the Middle Empire, the Sung dynasty (960–1126) was never able to bring about the reunification of China. But its political and military defeats fade before the importance of its technical and scientific progress (printing, the compass, gun-powder, mathematics and biology). At the end of the T'ang period the doctrine of the scholars, stifled by Buddhism and Taoism, was set on an upward course which was to reach its height with Chu Hsi (1130–1200). It was no exception to find an expert in many fields at once. For example, Shen Kua (1031–95) was architect, agronomist, doctor, historiographer and ambassador. He opposed the system of lunar months to the advantage of the solar calendar. He surmised, before Kepler, that the apparent course of the sun round the earth was elliptical and not circular, and he pointed out the exact position of the north pole. Pediatrics were elucidated by Ch'ien Yi (1023–1104), the greatest of Chinese pediatricians. He was the first to differentiate chicken-pox, measles, scarlet fever and smallpox. Preventive variolation was mentioned for the first time in 1014 by Wang Tan (957–1017), a prime minister of the Sung emperors. It was probably a foreign technique of Irano–Indian origin. Just as it was not highly esteemed by classical Arab medi-cine, so it was incorporated only at a late date into Chinese scien-tific medicine and for a long time was limited to popular practice.

Forensic medicine made its first appearance with the *Si-yuan-lu* (1247) of Sung Tz'u (1186–1249). The birth of forensic medicine coincides with a renewal of interest in anatomy following a

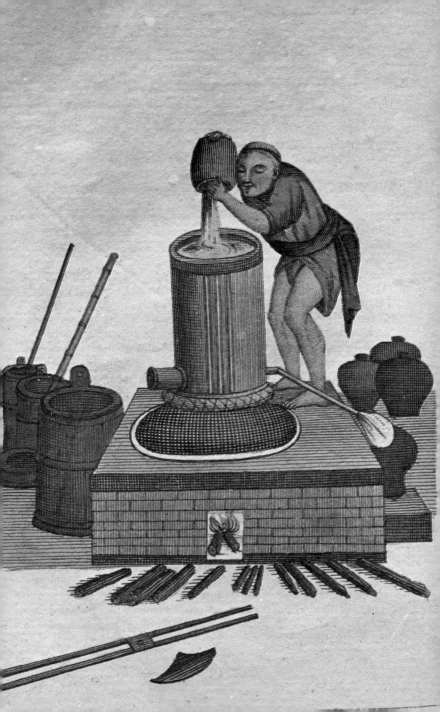

dissection in 1106, which we know through the drawings of Yang Chiai (*c*. 1068–1140).

The *materia medica* became highly developed and received the addition of many exotic drugs (mandragora, myrrh, theriac, fenugreek, opium, etc.). Progress here was linked with that of zoology and botany, and with South-Eastern and South-Western Asiatic connections.

Wang Wei-i (1026), doctor and sculptor, composed a compendium of acupuncture and cast two 'men of bronze' which were later frequently reproduced. They facilitated the location of acupuncture points.

For the first time collections of articles on medicine were checked, compiled and republished in encyclopedias printed from woodblocks and illustrated, sometimes in colour.

The Yüan dynasty (1260–1367) enjoyed the political domination of China but put her into close cultural relationship with the West. The Mongol expansion was accompanied by a sequence of devastation and destruction which reduced the population from one hundred million (*c*. 1125) to sixty million (1290), and there were also serious famines. Nevertheless a short time later Marco Polo (1254–1323) gave an account of a flourishing state, which was indeed at the furthest limit of its territorial aggrandisement, from Korea to Vietnam and from Japan to the Adriatic.

Under the Sui dynasty (581–617) the cultivation of the vine was intensified in Shansi province, and Egyptian experts came in order to perfect the manufacturing process of cane-sugar. Grain alcohol, obtained by distillation rather than by simple fermentation, became common in the thirteenth century and was introduced into medicine as well as into the drinks consumed by the Court. A Parisian goldsmith, Guillaume Boucher, built Kublai a mechanical fountain, surmounted by an angel blowing a trumpet, which provided the courtiers with rice-beer, wine, mead and koumiss. This implies a certain degree of alcoholism among the Mongol rulers. That the alcoholics were also debauched is to be gathered by studies of the genital organs by Yang Shih-ying (1264), who described genital 'chancres' associated with cephalic lesions. But there is no proof that these were cases of syphilis, nor even of venereal disease.

Yih-lu Ch'u-ts'ai (*ob.* 1243), one of Jenghiz Khan's greatest counsellors, saved many medical works from destruction. The Imperial College of Medicine was set up (1305) and a medical encyclopedia was reprinted (1300). Four famous names were associated with internal medicine: Liou Wan-su (*c.* 1120–1200), Chang Tzu-ho (*c.* 1156–1260), Li Tung-yuan (1179–1251) and Chu Tan-chi (1281–1358). Each had a pathogenic system which was to be the starting point for the later medical schools. Hu Szu-huei (*c.* 1314–30), an Imperial dietician, described deficiency diseases and their treatment by rational dietetics with no other medication.

Hua Shou identified the bluish-white spots which, appearing on the mucous membranes of the mouth, are the premonitory symptoms of measles; but he did not see their diagnostic value insisted upon by Flindt (1883), Filatov (1895) and Koplik (1896). He also revived the technique of acupuncture and was especially famous for his editions of the classics, such as the *Su-wen* of Huang Ti, the *Shang-han lun* of Chang Chung-ching and the *Nan-ching*.

The *Nan-ching* is a short work in two volumes comprising commentaries on eighty-one difficult passages taken from the *Nei-ching*. In addition it contains the first exposition of the theory of the pulse. It is not referred to in the Han Annals and is probably earlier than the time of the Three Kingdoms (220–65). The Sui and T'ang Annals attribute it to Pien Ts'io. It appears to be the work of compilers who lived under the Later Han dynasty (25 BC–AD 220). Lu Kuang, a Court Physician, is thought to have added a commentary composed in the third century. Ting To-tung and Yu Shu (both eleventh century writers) gave greater emphasis to physiology. They studied, for example, the course of the alimentary bolus (*shuei-ku*, water and grain) descending to the stomach where it is transformed into vapours (*ch'i*) by the action of the spleen. The bolus is then divided into impure and pure parts, the former being evacuated through the pylorus, the latter reaching the cardia where they become blood.

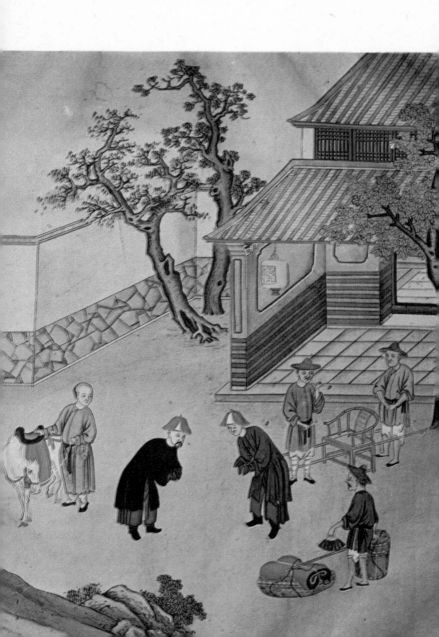

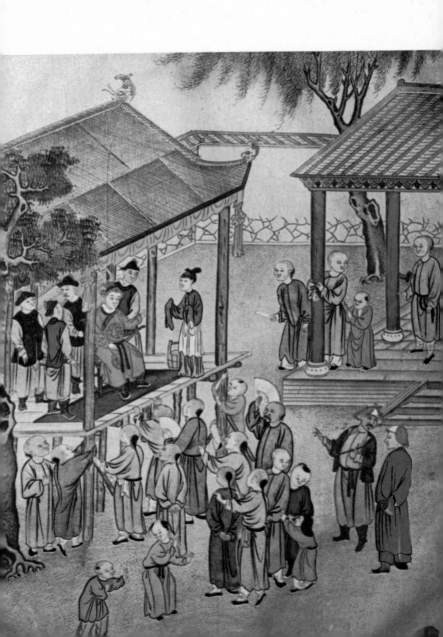

Hua Shou was the first to write a systematic commentary on the sphygmological part of the *Nan-ching*, and especially to define the contributions of the editors of the pre-Yüan period, on which he made exhaustive biographical and bibliographical notes: Su Tung-p'o (1036–1101), a doctor and scholar; Liou Wen-shu, the author of the *Ch'i-yun lun-o* ('The Circulation of the *ch'i*'), of the Sung dynasty (*c.*960–1126); P'ang An-shih (1042–99) who wrote the *Shang-han tsung-ping lun* ('Ailments Attributable to the Cold'); Chou Yu-chiuan, a Sung expositor of the obscure passages of the *Nan-ching* in the *Nan-ching pien-cheng shih-i*; Chi T'ien-si (*c.*1161–89), an editor of the *Nan-ching*, and others.

The established text of the *Nan-ching* with notes was probably compiled by Hua Shou in the twenty-first year of the reign of the Emperor Chih Chen (1361), and the text engraved in 1366. The original manuscript of the edition appears to have been lost. Chang Shih-hien produced another edition, printed between 1506 and 1521. Others are known, among them one by Shen Wei-yuan (1693).

The *Chu-chin t'u-shu tsi-ch'eng* ('Synthesis of Books and Illustrations of Ancient and Modern Times') compiled from 1701 to 1716 and printed in 1728, 1884–8 and 1890, still contained the text of the *Nan-ching*. A German version was produced by Hubotter.[13]

Irano–Arab medicine used Chinese texts and rhubarb; but with foreign practitioners Chinese medicine acquired Arab lapidaries, India chaulmoogra, opium and mandragora.

Modern Medicine

Thrust into power by a popular peasant revolution, the Ming dynasty (1368–1644) came between two foreign conquering dynasties, the Mongol and the Manchu. It freed Peking (for 432 years in the hands of barbarians) and, although Southernist, set up the capital there for the first time. In a kind of rediscovered golden age it was anxious to restore the intellectual and moral values of Chinese culture. The T'ang civilisation, considered to be the archetype, was frequently imitated, but a decline set in after Yung Lo (1403–24).

Contact with foreign medicine was made through the great voyages of the Imperial Fleet as far as West Africa (1405–24), the trans-Asiatic caravan trade and the arrival in Peking of Father Ricci (1601). It is important to note that at the time when Western medicine, brought by Ricci and his brother-Jesuits, was making contact with Chinese medicine, there was no phenomenon in the Far East comparable with the Renaissance in the West. There was no passing from a Gothic to a Promethean era, from universal and ideative concepts to nationalist and humanistic ones, from a feudal economy to capitalism.

The reasons for this are many and are not within the scope of this work. We must therefore confine ourselves to a rapid survey. By virtue of the formula, already commonplace in the third century BC, which divided the population into four classes: *shih* (scholars), *nung* (farmers), *kung* (artisans), *shang* (merchants), China was essentially a peasant society ruled by bureaucrats. For them the solution to all problems (even economic) was a moral one, since only by the perfecting of the self could the human order be aligned with the cosmic. By paralysing personal interest (*szu* and *li*) and the spirit of competition (*ching* and *ch'o*), the philosopher-politicians ruled out the creation of a mercantile, industrial and capitalist civilisation capable of suppressing the feudal régime and of providing a social and economic environment which would have favoured the development of science. Thanks to their control China has never had city-states, free cities, powerful guilds or mercantile maritime republics. They established a scale of values which was completely different from that of Western capitalists; hence an ever-growing discrepancy between the Western and the Chinese systems of evaluation.

With regard to the invasion of Far Eastern medicine by the medicine of the West, events took a completely different course in continental Asia (China and Vietnam) and insular Japan (cf. p. 78).

In China and Vietnam, Western medicine did not from a scientific

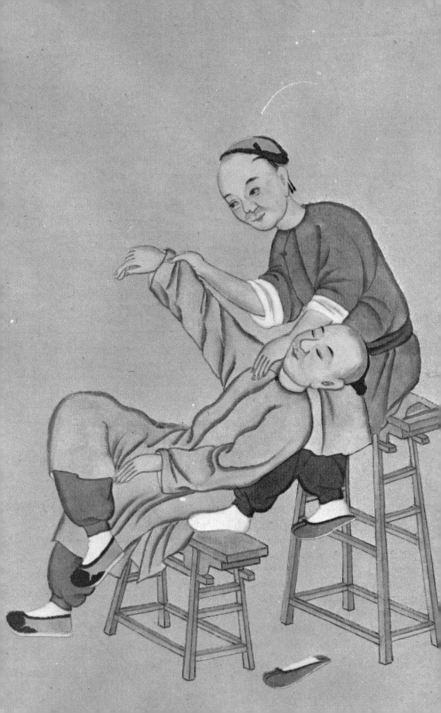

Pulse-taking during reanimation
of a patient. A water-colour made
on rice-paper, Ch'ing period.

49

point of view come to environments capable of receiving it. It was
for the use of the emperor alone that missionaries, themselves
strangers to the art of healing, compiled works in Manchu on
anatomy and the circulation of the blood. As these were written by
hand, relatively few copies existed and they seldom reached anyone
unconnected with the Court. Recognising the extent to which they
condemned traditional anatomy, the Emperor K'ang Hsi considered them to be of great interest for himself but dangerous for
his subjects. He fully realised that any break or displacement in the
closely-woven wickerwork of Chinese civilisation would disturb its
harmony and solidarity and was therefore to be avoided. The introduction of the teaching of Western medicine and allied sciences into
the Chinese educational system was thus fraught with danger.

Education was the blood and the veins (*hsiue-mo*) of the Empire.
'The law is a temporary curb. Only education can bind for ever,'
said K'ang Hsi. *Chiao* means in fact religion and education
together, and only a respect for the moral law could maintain a
social order implemented by a minute number of officials and a
sovereign who acted much more as an arbitrator over conflicts
than as a dictator. In view of this the State was less concerned with
the spread of knowledge than with the supervision of the competitive entrance to the public service. General education was much
less important than actual teaching, where reform was going
considerably beyond simple academic measures and was running
the risk of causing dangerous cracks in the already rotten Imperial
structure.

The only great scientific work written in the sixteenth century
outside the Western scientific influence of Copernicus, Vesalius and
Galileo is (as Needham says) the great *Materia Medica* of Li Shih-
chen (1518–93). It is the masterpiece of Ming medicine. Besides
being a great pathological and therapeutic work, it is a treatise on
natural history, giving a classification of mineral, vegetable and
animal products. To complete the encyclopedia there are chapters
on chemical and industrial technology and geographical, historical,
dietetic, culinary, cosmological, philosophical and philological

50

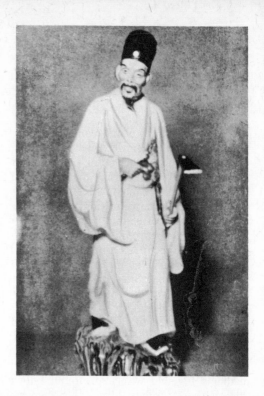

Li Shih-chen (1518–93),
author of the great Ming
dynasty encyclopedia and
materia medica.

data. It has been translated into all the languages of the Far East
and the principal Western languages. It mentions syphilis, which
appeared in China towards 1505–6 (more or less at the same time
as it was observed by Western, Arab and Indian doctors) and was
treated, as throughout Eurasia, by mercurial preparations and
China root.

Yang Chi-chou, also called Tsi-shih ('the saviour of his time'),
wrote on acupuncture. Born into an old family of doctors established in the Chekiang province from the T'ang period, he was, with
the great pharmacologist Li Shih-chen, the most famous doctor of
the Ming dynasty. He lived during the reigns of Shih-tsung (1522–
66) and Wan Li (1573–1619) but the dates of his birth and death are
not known. From an early age he had an omnivorous curiosity and
encyclopedic gifts. He first studied literature, but met with opposition and had to abandon it in order to be initiated into the
family art of medicine. His grandfather was a court physician

under the Ming dynasty. Yang Chi-chou had two sons, Ch'eng Cheng and Cheng Hiue. At the time of Shih-tsung, Yang Chi-chou was appointed official doctor (*I-kuan*) and acquired a great reputation. In 1568 he worked at the hospital of Shengtsi-Tien. In 1572 he lived in Peking, in the street of the River of Jade, and stayed there in official service during Wan Li's reign. But he was a great traveller: traces of certain of his famous treatments can be found in 1555 in Fukien province, in 1561 and 1562 at Lingtsi-Chung, and in 1580 at Yangchow. Out of compassion for his patients he went to the convent of Ngo-mei in 1572 in order to treat a friend suffering from typhoid. Similarly in 1574 he made a long journey to T'ien-t'an to cure the foster-father of another friend whose filial piety had moved him. In 1576 he went to Tsih-Chou and Yang-yin, where he stopped to visit the tomb of Pien-Ts'io. He also went to Shantung and, in the Shansi province, to P'ing-Yang.

On his travels he made innumerable notes which he meditated upon for forty-five years. He thus acquired an experience of rural medicine together with a profound knowledge of popular needs and of the customary drugs. He then started on the first three chapters of his work: 'Heaven, Earth and Man' (*Wei-sheng, Chen-chiou, Pi-yao*), to which Wang Chuo-chuang wrote a preface. It was the beginning of the *Chen-chiou ta-ch'eng*, which appeared later in the following circumstances: during the reign of Wan Li, the Imperial Censor Chao Wen-p'ing, Governor of Shansi, took one of his wonderful courses of treatment by three injections. With some help Yang Chi-chou reproduced the Medical College's *t'ung-jen* (copper model) and consulted more than twenty classics. He then wrote the ten chapters of the *Chen-chiou ta-ch'eng*; the engraving was begun in 1579 with the help of Huang Chen-ngan, and the first edition was published in 1601 at P'ing-Yang.

This great work is an encyclopedia of acupuncture which gives an excellent historical record of unwritten traditions as well as of the classics, condensed in short lines of rhythmic prose to assist the reader's memory. Family or personal recipes are edited in the same poetic style (the song of the conquering jade, the fire of the

Massage technique from
The Secrets of Massage
by Chou Yu-fan of the
Ming period.

volcano, the cold across the sky, the twitching of the dragon's tail, the swaying of the red phoenix's head).

Moreover the work contains exhaustive technical, clinical and therapeutic sections. The last chapter is devoted to pediatric diagnosis and massage therapy for children.[14]

Chou Yu-fan published a work (*T'uei-na pi-kiue*, 1573) on pediatric massage therapy. It was compiled by Chang Chen-chiun under the Ch'ing dynasty and republished at Peking (1956).

A real first-aid manual, it contains a section on symptomatology leading to diagnosis, and a therapeutic section comprising, in addition to physiotherapy exercises, the technique of fomentations, poultices, plasters, induced vomiting, medicinal baths, cauteries, moxas and acupuncture, not to mention amulets and incantations.

The ailments studied are: convulsions, cachexia, vomiting, diarrhoea, excess cold and heat, dysentery, fevers, coughs, suffocation, mumps, abdominal pains, jaundice, edema, tumours, bilious attacks, epilepsy, ophthalmia, umbilical tetanus, thrush, noma, ranula, sore throat and erysipelas. The author emphasises the peculiar features of pediatrics, called the mute's speciality (*a-ch'o*) because it is not possible either to question (*wen*) or to take the pulse (*tsie-mo*). Of the four classic points of examination there remain only inspection (*wang*) and audio-olfactive investigation, which require a great deal of intelligence (*shen*) and wisdom (*sheng*). As regards therapeutics, acupuncture is dangerous and medicines are brought up or badly tolerated. In many cases one must act quickly by external manipulation, for which the points of application and conditions are very precisely described. Comparable Japanese works were composed at the end of the eighteenth century under the generic heading 'treatment of urgent cases'.

Cases of traumatism, localised affections and general illnesses each had different areas for massage. In a general illness the massage of a particular area aimed at a specific effect usually at some distance from it. It might moreover be an acupuncture point, in which case the anticipated result would be comparable to the one acupuncture would produce. Each illness had theoretically its

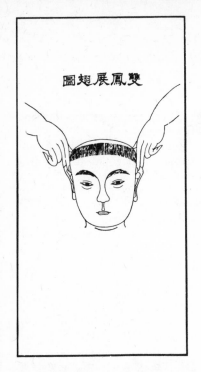

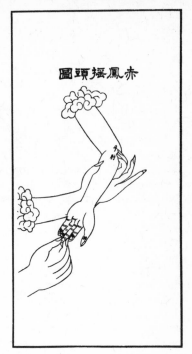

corresponding physiotherapy exercise. Massage was to be neither violent nor sluggish, neither light nor heavy. Sometimes it would fix (*ngan*), sometimes it would expel (*mo*). The masseur used the fleshy part of his fingers, the backs of his fingers or the whole palm according to the action required: he might dig in his finger-nail (*chia*), which would produce an effect similar to that of acupuncture, rub lightly with a circular motion (*jou*), push in a straight line and return (*t'uei*), pinch, push (*yun*), roll with both hands (*ts'uo*), shake (*yao*). Generally the bare hand was used, but it was sometimes considered useful to smear it with a preparation of onion and ginger or musk. There was no clear-cut distinction between the different procedures; they were completed and succeeded each other as occasion demanded.

Taoism still had an influence on medicine, as may be found in an anthology of Taoist works, the *Sing-ming kuei-che* (*c.* 1622). They divided the human body into three anatomical regions. The upper or cephalic region was the source of the spirits which

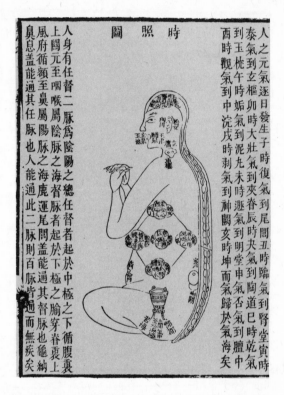

dwelt in the body. The pillow of jade (*yu-shen*) is situated low in the back of the head. The so-called pillow bone is the occiput (*shen-ku*). The palace of *ni-huan* (from the Sanskrit 'nirvana') is situated in the brain, which is called the 'sea of bone-marrow' (*suei-hai*). It was the source of the seminal essences.

The middle region was represented by the spine, which was not regarded as a functional column, but as a canal linking the cerebral cavities with the genitalia. It ended at a point called the 'celestial column' (*t'ien-shu*), at the hair line on the nape of the neck. It must

Taoist anatomy. *Left* This back view shows the genital organs (kidneys) communicating extensively, upwards, with the cerebral cavities through the spinal canal and, downwards, out through a spermatic duct. *Below* The side view shows a spermatic duct in front of the spine, which ensures the brain-kidney-exterior function. The two diagrams explain the technique of *coitus reservatus*, which directs the sperm to the brain (*ni huan*) and controls the physical body through the mind.

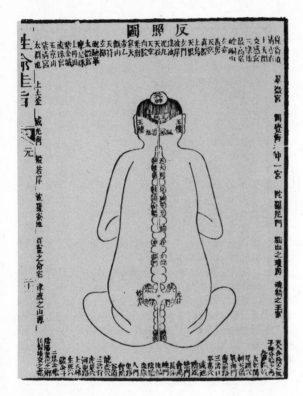

not be confused with the acupuncture point of the same name.

The lower region comprised the field of cinnabar (*tan-t'ien*) which will be referred to again later (see page 224). It was the seat of genital activity represented by the two kidneys: the tiger's fire (*yang*) on the left and the dragon's fire (*yin*) on the right. Sexual union was symbolised by a couple: a young man leading the white tiger and a young woman riding the green dragon. Lead (the male element) and mercury (the female element) were to mingle. Immediately they were united, the pair cast their essence into a bronze

Taoist gymnastics (*kung-fu*).
Breathing exercises and
meditation were essential
to inner well-being and to
longevity, according to
Taoist canons.

cauldron, the symbol of sexual activity. But instead of being excreted and lost, the genital fluids, particularly the sperm (*tsing*), were capable of returning to the brain by the vertebral column, which thus offered a means of following once again the 'path of life'. The basis of these Taoist sexual practices was *coitus reservatus*, during which the sperm which had descended from the encephalon to the bladder (but had not been ejaculated) returned to its source. This was called 'returning the essence' (*huan-tsing*). Whatever doubts we may have as to the reality of this return, it remains none the less true that the Taoists conceived a cerebral mastery of the basic instincts which kept the degree of genetic stimulation just below that of ejaculation. They thus brought to the sexual act a new technique and an end other than that of reproduction. Sexual practices played an important part in Taoism. Public, collective practices noted in the second century disappeared in the fifth. Private practices went on long enough for Ch'eng-tsu (twelfth century) to assign to them a section of his *Tao-shu*. Stripped of their religious content and adopted by doctors, they acquired a wide following under the banner of hygiene.[15] In actual fact both Taoist and Buddhist monks observed rules of continence. But the former regarded it as a form of detachment which was to lead them to deliverance, whereas the latter remained chaste so as not to have their energies dissipated, in order to concentrate, to retain their essence and to live for a long time. It is possible that the Taoists were inspired, as in the case of their breathing exercises, by Indian tantrist works, of which certain were translated into Chinese during the T'ang period and were known to Sun Szu-miao.[16]

The *Pao-p'u-tzu* contains a section entitled *The Bedroom* (eighteen chapters) which was printed in 1066 and reprinted in 1307, 1544 and 1604 by Chiao Shih-ning. Its data were reproduced on the basis of texts included in the Sui Annals by Tamba Yasuyori in his *I-sin-fang* (982–4) printed by Taki Genkin in 1854. This is a medical compendium in thirty chapters containing the 'Secrets of the Bedroom'. It was republished by Yih To-huei (1864–1927) who

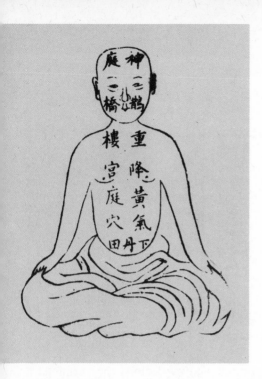
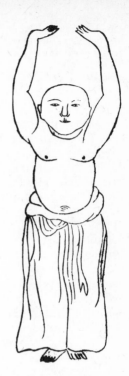

reconstructed the lost texts, in particular the *Ars Amatoria* of Tung Hiuan.[17]

The Ch'ing dynasty (1644–1911) was again a dynasty of foreign overlordship. But it was not tinged with that Syrio–Nestorian culture which had estranged the Yüan dynasty from the vast majority of their subjects and had made conditions favourable for its own downfall. Free of this blemish, the Manchus were to be tolerated for two hundred and fifty years and were to be able to repeat the Mongols' bid for universal power. Indeed they were sufficiently naturalised to establish themselves in Peking with the manifest desire of assimilation into the Chinese people. Despite fortunate beginnings they never succeeded in being adopted by the whole nation and they had almost incessantly to cope with Ming legitimists, nonconformist scholars, secret revolutionary societies, peasant risings, revolts by racial minorities and sea pirates. K'ang Hsi and Ch'ien Lung, two remarkable men, were followed (1795) by mediocre rulers who were crushed by the empire's increasing

Parallels between diseases and products of the three realms of nature (from Li Shou-sien's *Simple Study of Needles and Moxas* of 1798).

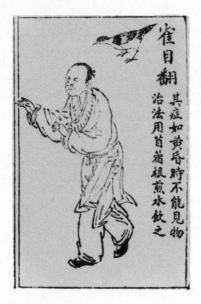
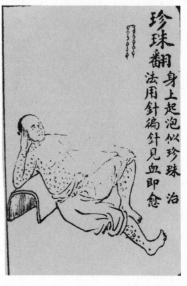

frailty, and were preoccupied with their attempts to deal with popular discontent and demands from abroad. The ultra-Chinese, feudalistic, equestrian, northernist, continental China was moreover gradually being overtaken by a southernist, pedestrian, maritime, commercial China which was already open to Western influence.

To the Ch'ing dynasty we owe the publication of great encyclopedias, published by Imperial Commissions, four times the size of the *Encyclopaedia Britannica* and containing medical sections. The compilation of ancient and modern books appeared in 1786, the Encyclopedia in Four Parts from 1772 to 1790. The Golden Mirror of Medicine (1739) was a third encyclopedia, illustrated, dealing exclusively with medical sciences. This was the time when, under the influence of protestant missionaries and doctors from the West, medicine in China, as in Japan, was invaded and conquered by

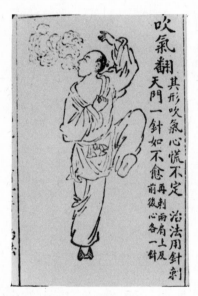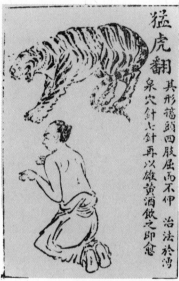

Western medicine, and when the importation of opium (the 'foreign poison', *yang-tu*) was imposed by 'unequal treaties'.

Several specialist works are worthy of note. The *Chen-chiou i-hiue* ('Simple Study of Needles and Moxas', 1798) by Li Shou-sien consists of three chapters, the last of which is devoted to a theory of 'signatures', seeking out analogical connections between illnesses and representations of the different natural kingdoms (animal and mineral). Four examples are:

1 Hemeralopia. This disease is likened to the difficulty of seeing at twilight, and it is treated with a draught prepared from lucern root. It is symbolised by a pigeon's eye.
2 General eruption of pearl-like pustules. They are treated by pricking with a needle until the appearance of blood indicates that they are cured.
3 Outbursts of anger symbolised by the 'exhalation of the breath'.

The heart-beats are irregular. *T'ien-men* acupuncture is used for treatment.

4 General contracture with stiffly-held head and all four limbs taut. It is treated by seven punctures of the *Yung-ts'iuan* point finished off with so-called realgar wine. It is symbolised by a savage tiger.

From 1784 to 1826 Chao Mai-ch'i (alias Chao Wen-tsin) compiled a work on surgery in which the exceptional wealth of instrumental equipment brings to mind the Tibetan or Indian stocks. It was clearly the fruit of long personal research by the author and explains certain operations carried out by the Chinese which had seemed impossible owing to the lack of appropriate instruments.

The work also contains an extensive and carefully prepared set of illustrations dealing particularly with dermatology and external pathology.

As early as the seventeenth century Chinese surgery was acquainted with cervical adenopathy, quinsy, tonsillar phlegmons, mastoid disease, and epithelioma of the lip. The *Sheng-ch t'u-chu hou-ch'o* (illustrated notes of symptoms and treatment in laryngology by Chang, 1822) studied the division between the buccal cavity and the pharynx. It was formed by the soft palate, the uvula, the tonsils and the back of the tongue which together constituted the throat (*yen-hou*). This area was the seat of seventy-two ailments, classified in a fundamentally descriptive way. The major functional syndromes (dysphagia, dysphonia, dyspnoea and coughing) were known. The work ended with articles on abscesses (*yin-chuang*) and several good descriptions of tumours of the throat, tongue (*shih*) and chin.

There were then under the Ch'ing dynasty specialists in laryngology well acquainted with quinsy and diphtheritic laryngitis. The treatment for these diseases consisted of: (i) a powder to be used locally, (ii) a potion, (iii) an appropriate diet.

The Dutch doctors of Batavia (Java) credited this treatment with an eighty per cent cure (A. Boddaert, Vorderman) and were availing themselves of it at the end of the nineteenth century.

At the beginning of this century it triumphantly withstood the invasion of antidiphtheritic serum.

During the Ch'ing the medical profession was organised in three streams: Court medicine, public medicine, and 'pavement' medicine.

The Court Medical College (also called the Imperial College or Imperial Academy of Medicine) was based on rules laid down by the Emperor K'ang Hsi. It consisted of the thirty or so doctors of the Imperial palaces, almost all of whom had a degree in the mandarinate, going generally from the copper button (ninth and lowest grade) to the crystal button (fifth grade). The highest in the hierarchy had to give periodic commentaries of the classics before their young colleagues who for their part had to be capable of consulting the twelve thousand works devoted to medicine and the natural sciences in the Imperial library. They also had to be able to draw up a prescription without smudges ·or touching up, impeccable in its presentation and calligraphy. This system was but a feeble image of its T'ang, Sung or Yüan predecessors. Indeed it cut a poor figure by the side of the Medical House of the Japanese *Shogun*. The first censor Wo Chang-yüan therefore submitted an unheeded supplication to the Throne dated 14 January 1866, requesting the reform of the Imperial College (*T'ai-i-yüan*) and strict examinations for its members.

Outside the Imperial palaces there was in existence a sketchy system of public assistance, the budget for which, financed partly by the State and partly by charitable organisations, was roughly half a million pounds in 1818. It was aimed at widows, orphans, the aged, and victims of drowning and disease. It provided the poor with wood and warm clothing in winter and a free coffin when they died. Its intentions were excellent but its funds extremely small. Charitable foundations, so numerous during the golden age of Buddhism, had lost all the importance they had under the Han, T'ang, and Sung dynasties. The interventions of K'ang Hsi and Yung Cheng had not saved them from their gradual decline.

The practice of private medicine began at the street-corner with soothsayers, geomancers, fortune-tellers and other purveyors of para-medical advice. It continued with ocularists, aurists, dentists, herbalists, cuppers and the barber-masseurs of whom Père Amiot has left a classic description. On a higher level there appeared the quack doctor who could be in one of several grades, from the most humble, setting out his remedies on the pavement, to the smartest, who would have an expensively and carefully arranged stall, either on a permanent pitch or on a movable cart. In the suburbs, bonzes and *tao-shih* practised in the shadow of the monasteries and distributed medical advice and amulets. These monk healers were in no way comparable to the lama-doctors of Mongolia or Tibet who had pursued complete courses of study in the medical institutes of the lama monasteries.

As soon as a patient had enough money he would put himself in the hands of either a doctor or an established pharmacist. Their emblem was a gourd (see facing illustration).

We have observed the efforts made by the great doctors of the earliest times to distinguish themselves from sorcerers and priests and to outclass them. Their victory was far from complete, and classical medicine, here as elsewhere, has never been able to eliminate occultism and magic completely. It even came to terms with them in several ways. The great works of the Middle Empire often assigned a place to incantations and charms, either in order to make allowance for public credulity or because they were acknowledged to have some efficacy. The same preoccupation can be found in contemporary Indian, Arab, or Byzantine writings. Just as Alexandre de Tralles (525–605) gave talismanic or mixed prescriptions, so did certain Chinese doctors.

They might also add to remedies of proven efficacy magical elements which would gradually oust in the patient's mind the purely medicinal part of the recipe. An example of this mixed therapeutic was to be found in the prescription (for certain forms of dyspepsia) of burnt paper, a yellow, very thick paper which produced a black, powdery ash containing charcoal together, doubtless, with mineral salts. On the paper, magic characters would

63

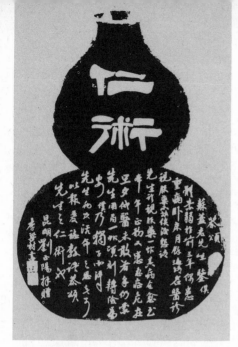

A gourd presented by a grateful patient to his doctor Su Kai. The inscription reads 'Being of a frail constitution, I contracted a serious illness three years ago and, confined to my bed for more than a month, I sought diagnoses from doctors everywhere. They gave me drugs with no effect until I asked the Master to examine me and to give me a prescription which overcame the illness,' etc.

be traced with coloured pencils composed of substances which in theory had medical properties. The red pencil contained mercuric oxide, the brown contained ferrous oxide, and the white contained calcium and magnesium carbonate. The patient had to consume the burnt paper and a few particles of the pencil mixed with hot water.

From the very earliest times there have been in Asia authoritative techniques which shaped or interpreted human destinies through numerical combinations and calculations. They have had a great success in China, where the connections between divination and medicine are many.

We may note the importance of propitious and unpropitious days indicated by special calendars for the application of medical and surgical therapeutic methods. Horoscopy and astrology would be used as bases for diagnosis or prognosis, often in conjunction with phrenology, physiognomy, palmistry and pedoscopy. Everything, even sphygmology, has been put to some divinatory purpose.

Yüan Liou-chuang (or Chung Ch'ih) compiled a work which was edited under the Sung dynasty by Chen Si-i. This was republished, notably in 1786, under the title *Shen-siang ts'iuan-pien* (complete treatise on the connection between the mind and the external features of the body), and is a classic on physiognomy. By observing the three parts (*san-t'ing*): forehead, nose and chin, and the five sensory organs (*wu-chuan*) together with other accessory features, the author deduces an individual's character, longevity and fortune. An organic failure can produce a change in the facial features, and in this way physiognomy has its occasional clinical usefulness.

To the Chinese, numbers are cyclic signs conceived to indicate position rather than order, and able to lead to combinations rather than totals. No wise man has ever consented to use them except where, without being forced into operations leading to an uncontrollable result, he could apply the knowledge to numerical games. Numbers have been used to express the qualities of certain groups (classificatory function), or to show an established arrangement (formalist function). The Chinese have therefore taken the greatest interest in the philosophy of numbers, but their numerical mental exercises have never led to the idea of quantity.[18] It is thus quite understandable that numerical divination should have influenced medicine, and it forms in fact the basis of the theories of the circulation of the blood and of ontogenesis.

Just as the stars circulate among the fifty celestial mansions in twenty-four hours, so the blood and the breath make fifty complete circuits of the body in the same space of time. The mythical value of the *yang* being nine, the square of that number gives the number of feet the blood will advance in a quarter of an hour, viz. eighty-one. A day containing a hundred quarters of an hour will give $81 \times 100 = 8,100$ feet. As the daily number of blood revolutions is fifty, the length of each revolution is $8,100 \div 50 = 162$ feet, viz. 81×2. It takes place in thirty minutes.

If eighty-one thousand inches are divided by the mythical value of the *yin* (six), this will give the number of breaths daily: $81,000 \div 6 = 13,500$. Since one breath corresponds to five pulse-beats, their daily number will be $13,500 \times 5 = 67,500$.

All female life is dominated by an odd number, seven. Teeth fall out and grow at seven months and seven years, puberty occurs at the age of fourteen and the menopause at forty-nine. Eight is the virile number, so that dentition has the two dates of eight months and eight years, puberty does not occur until the age of sixteen and the male climacteric is at sixty-four. At about this time (occasionally deferred until the age of seventy) sexual activity was considered to cease and the husband and wife could put together their clothes, which ancient ritual had hitherto required to be kept separate.

Similar ideas can be found in the work of Agrippa von Nettesheim (1486–1533). Starting from the figure seven, and with no sexual differentiation, he divided the human life into eleven stages: seven months, seven teeth; twenty-one months (3 × 7), beginnings of speech; thirty-five months (5 × 7), weaning; seven years, loss of first teeth; fourteen years (7 × 2), puberty; twenty-one years (3 × 7), marriageable age; thirty-five years (5 × 7), final cessation of growth; forty-two years (6 × 7), no further increase of strength; forty-nine years (7 × 7), beginning of senility; sixty-three years (7 × 9), climacteric; seventy years, normal span of life.

In his famous work on the abacus (*Suan-pan tsung-tsung*, 1593), Ch'eng Ta-wei demonstrated a mathematical process for determining the sex of the foetus during its intra-uterine life which is still very popular. Three factors come into play: the woman's age, the time of conception, and the moon (i.e. month). The last figure of the woman's age and that of the moon in which the pregnancy probably began must both be odd numbers for the child to be a male; if one is even and the other odd, the child will be a girl.

Whatever the importance of geomancy, numerical divination, physiognomy and other pseudo-sciences, they are at least to be found in a rationally motivated psychological context. We are now about to venture into a world where the classical categories of the mental mechanism lose all reality and are incapable of gaining any hold upon the powerful, obscure forces in the popular emotions. The impulsive attraction of the masses towards the miraculous and the supernatural was stimulated by certain deviationist forms of Taoism and Buddhism and by a popular religion in which more or

Talismans. These carried a special
form of writing, in the form of
rebuses with often cryptic meanings.
Left to right are talismans against:
palpitations, swellings, and eye ailments.

less secret societies and social, political, and Shamanist tendencies flourished. They cultivated states of trance, possession and emotional excitement, associated occasionally with social, religious, or sexual promiscuity. Such practices were called services of vice (*yin-szu*) in the Imperial decrees. To the Dionysiac attitude and excessive emotional excitement of the 'licentious' forms of worship the scholar civil servants were ordered (not always effectively) to oppose their Apollonian tendencies, based on the quest for the golden mean and a prudently balanced mental outlook.[19]

The two principal forms of magic are known in China: black, or aggressive, and white, or defensive.

Black magic, sometimes the cause of malignant anxiety-syndromes and even death induced by the suggestion of terror, did not develop in China to the extent observed in South America, Africa, Australia, New Zealand, the South Sea Islands and Haiti. Popular literature is nevertheless rich in stories of possession, in which 'vixens' (female were-foxes) take the form of a young woman in order to seduce travellers and cause them to die of consumption.[20] They have inspired a number of paintings, especially in Japan.

White magic attributes every disease or injury, every illness or disorder, and all strain to a diminution of the vital force in the human organism under the influence of a superior power. Hence the necessity for the use of extremely varied media in order to effect a cure: charms, prayers, exorcisms and incantations, drawings, talismans and medico-magical recipes. Processions, petitions to the gods, the widespread use of images of gods and spirits, offerings to tutelary spirits and pilgrimages were also advised. All these practices provided a livelihood for Buddhist and Taoist monks.

The bonzes came to the aid of the sick with invocations to the ten kings of the Buddhist hell (*shih-tien-yen-wang*), the famous *Kuan-yin*, the eighteen arhats, the patriarch Huei-nang, founder of the sect of herb-eaters and the healing saint, P'u-Ngan (*c.*1170).

Taoist talismans date back to Chang Tao-ling, the first official leader of Taoism, who was called the 'Master of Heaven' (*T'ien-shih*). At Lung-hu-shan (Kiangsi) he composed a book of talismans

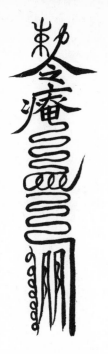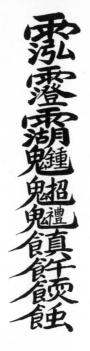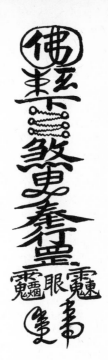

to cure the sick (*c.*126–145). Père Doré has classified them as follows:

1 Therapeutic talismans, of general efficacy or, on the other hand, useful only for a given disease of physiological condition (childbirth).
2 Substitute talismans (*t'i-jen*), figurines to which the patient's ailments would be transferred.
3 Talismans against demons, having the power to expel the malignant spirits causing the disease.
4 Lucky talismans, working as preventives before the appearance of the disease.

The vehicle for the talismans, a substantial feature of modern Taoism, was a white, red or, more frequently, yellow paper, yellow being the Imperial colour. It would bear a special kind of writing, governed by secret formulas and rules. Certain stylised characters formed rebuses of very difficult interpretation, but they were only rarely masterpieces of calligraphy. At all events Chinese talismans drew all their strength from the characters they bore.

A talisman against the 'five venomous animals' (the viper, scorpion, scolopendra, toad and spider). It is surmounted by the character *ch'ih* ('Imperial order', 'order patent') comprising the element 'strength' (*li*) which is placed above the *t'ai-chi* and the eight trigrams (*pa-kua*).

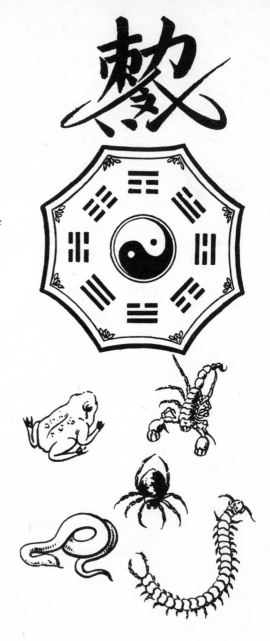

Ideographs, much more than alphabetic writing, have always held a magical, poetic power and have fascinated the imagination of the masses by evoking the acts, objects, ideas and feelings denoted by their graphic symbols.

Calligraphers may be classified as capable (*neng*), excellent (*miao*), inspired (*shen*), nonconformist and unrestrained (*i*).

The truly inspired calligrapher works

in a completely dispossessed condition, vibrant in his harmony with the world, withdrawn into the very heart of nature. He dissociates himself from human stupidity and is lost beyond the sun and the moon in a dazzling world where dullness is vanquished and death impossible. (Nicolas–Vandier.)

The human hand, the wind or the water turning the written formulas in a wheel are not praying but simply setting in motion the ritual energy contained in the printed characters. In the same way, by virtue of the power and authority which they signify, these sigillate or related characters have in the end acquired the gift of healing the sick. Thus, seals cut from official documents have been used as local remedies on ulcers or wounds.

Messages to the celestial or infernal powers have been used in the treatment of the widest possible range of illnesses. The phraseology of these invocations varies: a simple wish, involving only the writer, an impersonal order given in the name of the three religions, (*san-chiao*), or a command from the Buddha himself or some other supernatural personage.

In 1910 the authorities at Pakhoi used fireworks, fastings, the prohibition of the slaughter of domestic animals, and religious ceremonies in their efforts to combat the plague. Public collections covered the expense of these demonstrations and paid for a well-known doctor to come from Canton to reassure the inhabitants. Such a mentality did little to help orthodox medicine in its struggle against epidemics. The necessary health precautions, certification of death, inspection and autopsy of corpses, and destruction of contaminated huts were taken as so many futile and unacceptable irritations by people who attributed the scourge to supernatural causes. Their resentment was focused upon the European doctors who had undertaken the fight against the diseases. Parallel demonstrations were observed at the time of the plague epidemic in the Chinese quarter of San Francisco (1900–04).

In Imperial China, at once so near and so far from us, the government did not combat epidemics by appealing to its own official medical establishment. Paradoxically, and for all their rationalist Confucianism, the high civil servants resorted to magic practices.

During the plague epidemic which struck Mengtsz in 1896 the *Taotai* assembled the soldiers of his guard each evening in front of his *Yamen* and made them fire salvoes in all directions to frighten the demon of the plague.

At Yunnanfu, Governor Tsen gave orders for the city gates to be closed and the armed garrison to be assembled. The men were then marched towards the south gate, each soldier striking invisible demons with his sabre. A furious charge through the opened gate ended this symbolic massacre.

In 1895, at the time of the cholera in Peking, inscriptions of this kind were to be seen on the houses: so-and-so who lives here has burnt more than eleven taels' worth of gunpowder in honour of the *Kuei* of the epidemic.

During the bubonic plague at Canton (1893–4), the Cantonese held their new year celebrations during the sixth and seventh moons in an attempt to make the spirit of the disease think that he had mistaken the time he had chosen. At the same time Yersin was isolating the plague bacillus.

In other cases a pagoda might be built in order to ward off an epidemic. Here we have the idea of *feng-shui* (geomancy) which, by acting upon a point precisely determined by the geomantic compass, could turn away evil influences.[21]

The town of T'ung-chou, terminus of the great canal near Peking, requested that the Peking-Tientsin railway, opened in 1897, should not come and disturb their dead and so expose them to the risk of epidemics.

There is therefore nothing surprising in the fact that the Boxer movement (*I-ho ch'üan*, 'Fists of Justice and Harmony'), which also took the name *Shen-ch'üan* ('Boxers Helped by the Gods'), was a movement at once xenophobic and religious in which 'perverted practices' played an important part. Charms and incantations were regularly used both for the curing of disease and to endow the fighters with invulnerability.

Technical accomplishment in hypnotic procedures (*ts'uei-mien-shu*), in suggestion (*ngan-shih*) and, perhaps, in trickery gave rise to spectacular phenomena of trances, possession, catalepsy and emotional excitation on the part of the boy-mediums. The exhibitionist displays convinced the public that the Boxers held a 'commission from heaven'.[22]

The Boxer episode marked the end of a medieval period of xenophobia and magic which was to be replaced by a deconsecrated, secularised nationalism concerned only with immediate social and national demands.

2 Chinese Medicine and the Medicine of other Asiatic countries

All the states surrounding China (formerly called tributary states) have their popular aboriginal medicine which is the relic of a very ancient cultural substratum, some of the ethnic groups from which it comes being already extinct. It is to be contrasted with a scientific medicine recorded in writing and coming sometimes from exclusively Chinese, sometimes from Indo-Iranian sources.

In Korea, Japan, and Vietnam, the origins of scientific medicine can be traced to a common shared source as well as to China. Although the basic doctrines take a Chinese form, they are not the same as those of the Chinese classics. In their conception of illness and therapeutics some doctors in the three countries were able to preserve the same originality and critical outlook as were Arab doctors vis à vis the Greek tradition or Western doctors vis à vis Graeco-Latin and Judaeo-Arab opinions. By virtue of this, they long ago acquired a by no means negligible position in the evolution of Chinese medicine.[1]

At the end of the nineteenth century Chinese medicine was partially eclipsed by the medicine of the West, even in the countries where from time immemorial it had been the only science of any standing. The liberation of continental China and the decolonisation of South-East Asia were accompanied by the revival of this traditional medicine in all countries which had been open to Chinese influence. Today, as in the past, the masses turn to ancient therapeutic methods which can still be of considerable use if corrected in the light of contemporary medicine, and which are to be commended for their moderate cost.

Korean Medicine

As early as the Chou dynasty cultural exchanges took place between Confucian, pre-Buddhist China and Korea. Korea also played an important part in the transmitting of Chinese medicine to Japan. Doo Jong Kim (1958) has given a good account of the working of these exchanges and their influence on books, medicines, and men. Korean doctors gave the Chinese data a personal note and added Indian data which they had received from Buddhist missionaries.

From the fifth to the eighth century, Korean magician-healers, herbalist apothecaries, and doctors were on several occasions responsible for the care of Japanese rulers. Later, the Japanese dispensed with this intermediary by sending their students to China direct or by bringing over Chinese masters. Korean sources were nevertheless still in use for a long time and well-stocked libraries were formed containing precious works which were no longer to be found in the countries of their origin. There was the famous work on essential plants, *Pen-ts'ao*, of the Shao-hing period (1159), brought back as spoil by Ukita Hideye at the time of Toyotomi Hideyoshi's expedition (1592). This extremely rare book, with text and drawings in their entirety, is preserved at the Kyoto Botanical Garden.

The Koreans are very proud to belong to the oriental cultural tradition (*Tong-hak*), but unfortunately the Korean medieval period remains more or less unknown to Western historians.[2] The Korean scholar's language in both history and medicine is Chinese, and the first texts deal with the transmission of Korean medicine to Japan.[3] Fragments from Chinese medical classics were first introduced about AD 200. Kwan Rok (Kwanroku in Japanese), a bonze and doctor at Paikze during the period of the Three Kingdoms, came to Japan in 602 to teach the medical art of the mainland. A Japanese acupuncture specialist, Kihabenkinama, went to Shilla to win for himself the degree of Doctor of Acupuncture. The record of these exchanges is preserved in extracts of works, the *Paikze shin chip bang* ('Anthology of Paikze Prescriptions') and the *Shilla Bup Sa Bang* ('Prescriptions of the Masters of Shilla'), the originals of which are lost. These prescriptions are mentioned in the Japanese work by Tamba Yasuyori (*I-shin-ho*, 984), (Chinese: *I-sin-fang*), a summary of Chinese classical medicine. This book was inspired in its essentials by the work of Sun Szu-miao and the famous 'Treatises on the Bedroom'.

Among the most important Sino-Korean works mention should

Two illustrations from the *Chi Jong Ji Nam* (*c*. 1500). This important Sino-Korean work on the treatment of abscesses is attributed to Im Eun Kuk. It recommends cures by acupuncture.

be made of the *Hyang-yak Ku-gup-bang*, probably composed in the middle of the thirteenth century; the first and only copy known in Japan dates from 1417. It deals with the medical use of the local fauna and flora. The remedy most in demand was the famous Korean ginseng. The *Hyang-yak Chip Sung Bang*, published in the fifteenth year of the reign of Sejong (1433), classified 10,706 recipes which eventually spread to Japan. But in the fifteenth century the problem of such exchanges in a region which used Chinese as its sole working language was complicated by the invention of Korean transcription. Sejong ordered the Court Physicians and medical officials to produce an encyclopedia containing the classical prescriptions of all periods from the Han to the Ming. It was entitled 'Collection of Classified Medical Prescriptions' (*Ui Bang Yoo Chui*, 1445), and the only copy known is also in the possession of the Japanese Imperial Household. Other editions, providing an excellent introduction to the history of early medicine in China, are reproductions of 1852. The *Chi Jong Ji Nam* (*c*.1500) is less famous. It is a 'Compass for the Treatment of Abscesses' and is basically confined to external pathology. It specifies the treatment of crucial abscesses by acupuncture and includes observations on tympanites, lumbar pains, asthma, etc. It is attributed to Im Eun Kuk, a doctor who lived during the reign of Chung Jong (see facing illustration). But the most popular Korean writer was Huh Joon, the author of the 'Golden Mirror of Oriental Medicine' (*Tong ui po kam*, 1613).[4]

Japanese Medicine
In 561–2 Chi Chung, a doctor from southern China, took to Japan more than a hundred books on theoretical medicine, acupuncture, and moxibustion which became the primer of classical medicine (*Chia-i ching*). As early as 608 E-Nichi and Fu-ku-in studied medicine on the mainland for fifteen years, afterwards returning home to spread the knowledge of Chinese medicine. A century later Japan took as its models the institutions of the T'ang Empire.

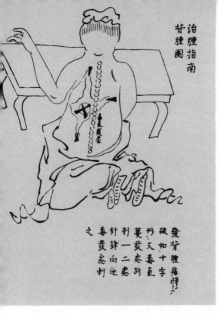

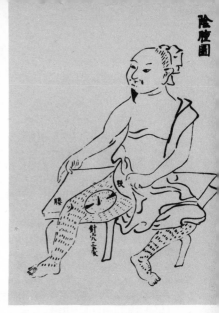

The Code of the Taiho period (702) controlled medical studies, the categories of specialisation and the membership of the Academy of Medicine and the provincial colleges.

In the Nara period (710–84) several Sino-Korean bonze-doctors crossed to Japan to teach Buddhism and medicine, among them being Kan Jin (687–763) who landed in 755. The following year the Emperor Shomu died, whereupon the Empress Komyo presented more than six hundred precious objects, some of which had been the Emperor's personal property, to the Todaiji temple. Together with these objects was a stock of sixty medicines, beautifully labelled, for the use of poor patients. They are still preserved in the Todaiji-Shosoin which is one of the earliest wooden buildings in existence and one of the oldest museums in the world. They have all been identified and their position noted in the works on *materia medica* of the T'ang (618–907) and Sung (960–1279) periods. From that time onwards there was no Chinese classic which the Japanese did not know and value. Special mention may be given to the two parts of the 'Classic of Internal Medicine' (*Nei-ching*), the *Materia Medica* ascribed to the legendary emperor Shen Nung (*Shen Nung pen-ts'ao*), 'Ailments Attributable to the Cold' (*Shan-han-lun*, c.217), and Ch'ao's work on etiology and pathology (c.610).

Ch'ao Yuan-fang's work on etiology (*Ch'ao-she ping-yuan*, 610) and Sun Szu-miao's 'Thousand Costly Recipes' (*Ts'ien-chin-fang*) were put into Japanese. During the Heian period (784–1186) a reaction in underlying local elements marked a set-back in Chinese influence parallel with the crumbling of the T'ang dynasty, but that this influence remained important is symbolised by the voyage of the monk Ennin during the reign of the Emperor Wen-tsung (827–40). Herbalists composed Sino-Japanese glossaries (*Honzo-wamyo*) and the lexicographer Minamoto No Shitagau (911–83) produced a dictionary of medical terms borrowed from Chinese (*Wamyosho*). The *Honzo-wamyo* were inspired in the main by the great *Materia Medica* of the T'ang period (*T'ang pen-ts'ao*). They gave plant names in very archaic regional dialects, long forgotten in China, and are therefore of considerable linguistic interest.

Tamba Yasuyori (912–995), known for his *Ishin-ho*, wrote an account of the Buddhist theory of the four elements. Among his sources were the 'Classic of Internal Medicine', Ch'ao Yuan-fang's book on etiology and pathology, Sun Szu-miao's 'Thousand Costly Recipes' and parts of a lost work on pharmacology (*Sinshu Honzo*) taken from the *Sin-siou-pen-ts'ao* by Su Ching (254 drugs). This last work is known only through the quotations studied in the *Ishin-ho*, as is also the *Yaikkei Taiso*.

During the Kamakura period (1187–1333) many new Buddhist sects flourished, and with them bonze-doctors such as Yurin (1362–7). The Zen sect is interesting for its close connection with the development of medicine, poetry and the arts. Of Chinese origin, it played a part in disseminating the respiratory techniques and the judo and karate elaborated on the mainland. Through the sects the Sung classics became the intermediaries for those of the T'ang period and thus continued to provide the foundation of Japanese medicine. The majority of books were still written in Chinese, but a few were phonetically transcribed into Japanese characters and others were completely translated. The *Manan-ho* (*c.* 1314), a collection of prescriptions compiled by Kajiwara Shozen, was inspired by Sung medicine, namely the Chinese work on the three causes of disease by Ch'en Yen (*c*.1161). But Kajiwara did not hesitate to criticise his masters on the mainland when he considered it appropriate. Monk-doctors were still to be found in large numbers during the Muromachi period (1336–1568), many travelling in the Yüan and Ming empires. Sanki Tashiro (1465–1537) founded the school of Li and Chu which propagated throughout Japan the teaching of the two famous doctors of the Sung and Yüan periods: Liou Wan-su (*c*.1120–1200) and Chu Tan-chi (1281–1358). Liou traced the principal cause of disease to an excess of *yang* (likened to animal heat). Chu devised the theory of internal fires in pathogenic conflict. His second hypothesis was the *yin-yang* conflict, in which the latter element always predominates. In its Japanese version this teaching minimised the traditional importance of the *pneuma*, disorders of the 'entrails' (*fubyo*) and ailments caused by cold (*shokan*), and emphasised external and internal factors. The former accounted for disturbances in the principal organs, while the latter would transmit the cause of the disease to the vascular system. The best known works of Li Tung-yuan, alias Ming-chih (1180–1251) are his book on practical medicine and surgery (*Nei-wai shang-pien huo-lun*), a work on the spleen and the stomach (*Pi-wei-lun*) and a summary of the treatments of five classics (*Wu-ching chih-fa chi-yao*). The most widely read Chinese works are a book on the circulation of the breath (*Yun-ch'i yao-chih lun*) and the 'Compendium of Medicine' (*I-fang tsing-yao*) by Liou Wan-su (*c*.1120–1200), a work on the natural sciences (*Ko-chih yu-lun*) by Chu Tan-chi (1281–1358), 'Doctors' Methods' (*I-chia ta-fa*) by Wang Hao-chu (1297), 'Summary of Therapeutics' (*Shih-i to-hiao-fang*) by Wei I-lin (*c*.1337), etc.

The Azuchi-Momoyama period (1569–1615) covered less than half a century, but its importance lies in the introduction of Western science to Japan by the Portuguese and the foundation of the Medical School of the Southern Barbarians (*Namban igaku*). It was moreover at this time that Confucianism superseded the Buddhist philosophy.

Dosan Manase (1507–94) was the leader of the Li-Chu school. A convinced Confucian, he worked towards the expulsion of bonze-doctors from the profession and their replacement by secular practitioners. He was a whole-hearted supporter of acupuncture and moxibustion (*Shinkyu Shuyo*). Tokuhon Nagata (1512–1630) was an opponent of the classical Chinese school. The Chinese works studied were still those by Chu Tan-chi (1281–1358) which specialised in *yin* tonics (*Chuan-i pu-yin wei-tsung*), or 'Tan-chi's Methods' (*Tan-chi sin-fa*). Wang Lun's commentaries on the Ming doctors (*c.*1502) still featured, and the famous *Materia Medica* revised in the Shao-hing period (*Shao-hing chiao-ting ching-shih cheng-lei pei tsi pen-ts'ao*) was known by the Japanese title *Shoko kotei keishi shorui bikju Honzo*. It had a profound influence on the Japanese school and was given a fresh set of illustrations (*Rukyo hongo*) drawn by naturalists.[5]

The Yedo period (1616–1867) saw the prosperous development of the so-called 'southern barbarian' or Dutch school of European surgery (*Namban-ryu-geka* or *Oranda-ryu-geka*). But the triumph of Western medicine was far from sounding the death-knell of the Chinese school. At the very time when the Japanese were showing an enthusiasm for Western medicine (at the cost of an amazing technical and linguistic effort) they still had a particular affection, at once very eclectic and very objective, for their masters on the Chinese mainland. Without renouncing anything of their ancient character, they wished to assimilate Western science just as they had already absorbed Indian Buddhism and Chinese culture. The conditioning of the Japanese to Indo-Chinese culture was in fact such that, even if they had desired it, they would have found it impossible to change their system of reasoning. Only to the extent that the science of Asia appeared obsolete were they able to try to replace its outdated values with efficient Western ideas and keep their own soul. They thus arrived at a carefully contrived syncretism which brought together Eastern traditions and Western progress.

Whilst they borrowed an unknown anatomy and surgery from Europe they remained largely dependent on China in many fields,

The extraction of a foetus,
head last, by Teizo Kondo.
From the Japanese *Atlas
of Obstetric Operations*
(*Tassei-zusetsu*), *c*. 1858.

79

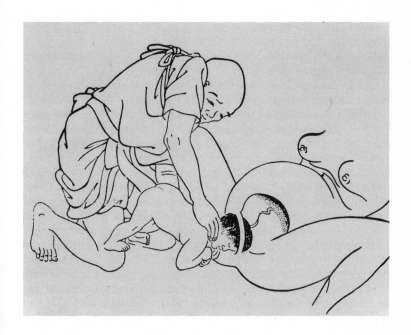

notably in teaching. As in China, there were many medical schools. Besides the Li-Chu school there was the one inspired by Chang Tzu-ho (1156–1260) (its Japanese name was the Schiwa Chos school), which was patronised by Toan Aiba (*d*. 1674). It attributed disease to disturbances in the circulation of the breath (*ch'i*) descending from the sky. The *Ko-I-Ho* or *Ko-I-Do* school (former true school of medicine) originated with Gen-i Nagoya (*d*. 1696). An enthusiastic student of logic, he wished to bring about in the field of medicine a movement parallel to that of the Han school (*Han-hiue*) on the mainland and to return to original sources. Just as the neo-Confucianist philosophies of Chu Hsi (1130–1200) and his adversary Wang Yang-ming (1472–1528) were to be abandoned in favour of the authentic thought of Confucius, so the

The crab (*hiai*). From a
Japanese album of materia medica
edited by Baron Cuvier.

Sung medical systems were to be rejected and replaced by the great classics of antiquity; thus Chang Chung-ching's 'Fevers' or 'Ailments Attributable to Cold' was known in Japanese by the title *Sho Kan-ron*.

The opinions of Gonzan Goto (1659–1733), the founder of the *Ikki-Ryutai-Ron* school, were in line with this tradition. He held that cold, wind, heat and humidity could restrict the circulation of the *pneuma* and lead to its stasis in certain parts of the body. Toyo Yamawaki (1706–63) and Shuwan Kagawa (1683–1755) were the main exponents of this theory.

Whatever their doctrinal divergences, these schools diagnosed diseases by inspection of the tongue, abdominal examination and the sphygmology of Wang Shu-ho's (*c.*210–285) *Mo-ching* and Li Shih-chen's book on the eight azygous veins.

Variolation, known in China as early as the twelfth century, was not brought to Japan until 1652–4 by a Chinese refugee, Sai Mun-cho, whose pupils were Masanoa Ikeda and his grandson Zuisen Ikeda (1734–1816). Acupuncture and moxas had already been mentioned in the *Ishin-ho*, but it was not until Dosan Manase and Gonzan Goto, who recommended polymoxibustion for serious illnesses, that they really became important. Waichi Sugiyama (1610–94) founded a school which lasted from 1681 to 1871. During his time, gold and silver needles were used in Japan instead of the Chinese steel needles. The needle was no longer inserted into the dermis by hand but with a little hammer or tubular punch. With this technique of tubular insertion Sugiyama cured the *shogun* Tsunayoshi Tokugawa of a serious illness.

There were two methods of locating acupuncture points: first the classic 'men of bronze' descended from Chinese prototypes and in new versions resulting from the collaboration of doctors, sculptors and bronze-founders; then dolls made of wood (see p. 83) or papier mâché, of which there is a good example in the museum of medical history of the Paris *Faculté de Médecine*. A more interesting venture was made towards a better knowledge of the external morphology of the human body, a subject which

○うみ蟹　雄蟹螂　雌
　　　　　　　　　博帯

郭索　無腸公子

海河川津山石の間
数種あり
　　　　　　猶溪

うちくれ蟹もおよぶの
　　　　　　　　撚祖

麋のもよあふまた
　　あつ〲
　　嘘のそくきせ
　　　　　英軺

沢蟹独舟ふりくねまづを
　　　　　　　　　萁より

82

Right Resuscitation
by facial manipulation.
Two pages from the 'First Aid'
(*Kokeisai Kyuho*) of Rankei Taki
published in three volumes
in 1789.

developed under the stimulus of the introduction of Western anatomy and enjoyed considerable success. It was at this time that some Japanese students raised doubts about the existence of the 'meridians', and others attempted to account for acupuncture with the help of European data. The Japanese methods of acupuncture and moxibustion were known in Europe through the work of Wilhelm Ten Rhyne (*c.* 1649–1700), Engelbert Kaempfer (1651–1716) and Peter Thunberg (1743–1828). It was Kaempfer who brought the words *moxa* (from the Japanese *mogusa*) and *moxibustion* into the European vocabulary.

At all periods the Chinese *Pen-ts'ao* and similar works were almost all translated and edited in Japan after a lapse of one or two centuries. The Edo period was no exception, even seeing the reappearance of the Korean intermediary.

In 1592, one year before Li Shih-chen began publishing his *Pen-ts'ao chang-mu*, Toyotomi Hideyoshi's troops brought back from Korea, as we have already seen, the famous *Shao-hing pen-ts'ao* with its coloured wood-engravings, all the Chinese editions of which have been lost. This book excited great interest in Japan. It was translated with the title *Honzo komoku* and was republished many times after 1596. Its fifty-two chapters dealt with the study of over a thousand plants and over a thousand animals.

The first appearance of the *Pen-ts'ao chang-mu* (1593) in Japanese translation (*Honzo komoku*) may be put at 1627. This famous work was the subject of many Japanese compilations and translations (see the authors' own bibliography (1957)). Hiraga Gennai (1729–79) still used Li Shih-chen's classification in his study of the products of nature (1763).

Chinese forensic medicine was still held in high regard. Naohisa Kawai followed Chinese models in his *Muben-roku-jutsu* in 1736. He was naturally acquainted with the *Si-yuan-lu* ('On the Redress of Injustice') written by Sung Tz'u, a Superintendent of Justice during the reign of Li Tsung (seventh year of the Shun-you era, 1247). Sung had been first initiated into the neo-Confucianism of

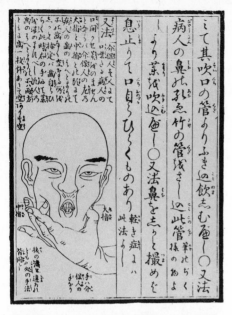

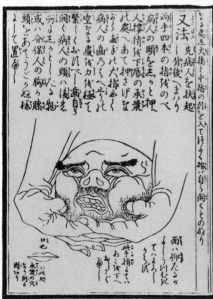

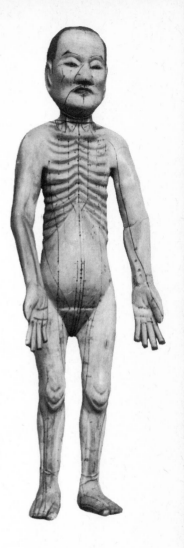

Above Japanese anatomical model for the study of acupuncture (nineteenth century).

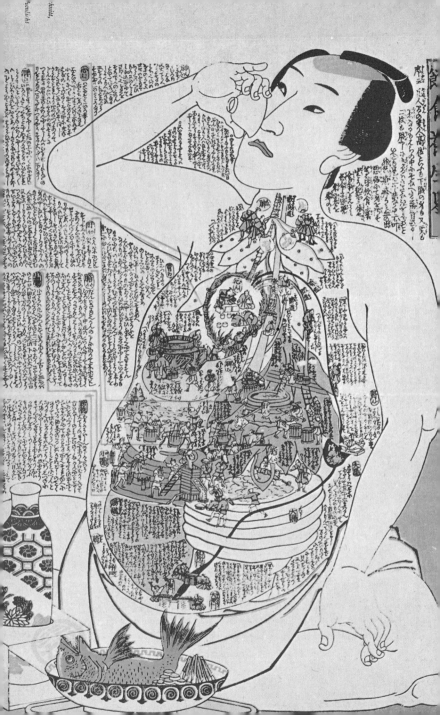

Left 'The mirror of eating and drinking', a Japanese colour engraving attributed to Utagawa Kunisada (1786–1865), dated about 1850. It illustrates the physiology of digestion according to Chinese and Japanese theories.

Below The Japanese actor Ichikawa Ebizo in the part of a travelling apothecary at the Ichimura-za theatre. The background is covered with inscriptions in theatre characters: the monologue of the apothecary praising his wares.

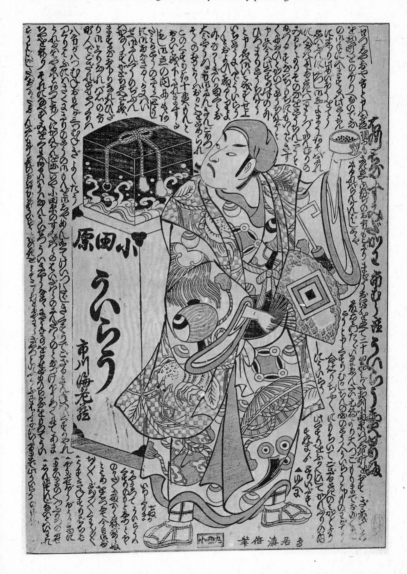

Chu Hsi by his masters Wu and Chen and had been promoted to the rank of 'Accomplished Scholar' in 1217. He was appointed administrative officer at Kanchow and subsequently became the Superintendent of Justice in Canton and Hunan and eventually Inspector-General.

The original manuscript of the *Si-yuan-lu* consisted of only two chapters. Then, under the Yüan dynasty, in the eighth year of the Ta-to era during the reign of Ch'eng-tsung (1304), six anatomical charts were added for the purpose of defining wounds: three charts (two front view and one back) locate the sixteen frontal and the six dorsal vital points, and the thirty-six frontal and twenty dorsal non-vital points. These areas, marked in red or black, 'restrict life'; hence the name 'vital points'. Another chart presents a detailed description of the skull, and the collection is completed by two osteological charts (front and back views). Under the Ch'ing dynasty, in the thirty-third year of the reign of K'ang Hsi (1694), the Institute of Law produced a version entitled *Wu-yuan-lu* which in 1770, during the reign of Ch'ien Lung, was illustrated with new osteological charts. Many subsequent editions (1777, 1796, 1827, 1831, 1854, 1876, 1891) under different titles testify to the great success of this work. The 1694 version was the one chiefly used by Naohisa Kawai.

In the twentieth century the medicine of China still occupies an important position in Japan. Its history does not fail to arouse considerable interest and there are traditional institutes which still live by 'Chinese Medicine'. The study of the *pen-ts'ao* has developed extensively. At the end of the nineteenth century Yamanashi and Nagaï isolated ephedrine (1885) from the famous remedy advocated by Chang Chung-ching (*c.*163–217) in his work on fevers. This was *Ma-huang* (*Ephedra sinica*). Research of this kind has continued uninterrupted at all levels.

The Society of Oriental Medicine (*Toyo Igaku-kai*) with corresponding members in Vietnam, is principally interested in *materia medica*, together with acupuncture. Since 1911, both subjects have been studied afresh to Western standards and by

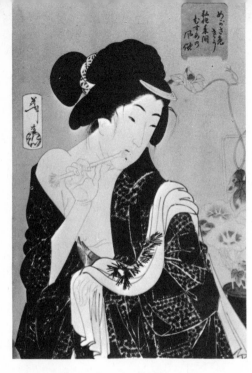

Japanese woman brushing her teeth. A nineteenth century engraving from an unknown source.

experimental methods. The increase in the number of blood corpuscles has been observed by Seikoku Aochi, Shimetaro Hara, Joichi Nagatuya, Hideji Fujii and Bunjiro Terada. The possible increase of complements and other antibodies by Seikoku is the subject of research by Aochi and Kaoru Tekieda. Hyperalkalosis of the blood and of the bones has been observed by Hisashi Kurozumi and Shigeroto Mizuno.

Mitchio Goto has drawn attention to the intensification of intestinal peristaltism and Kazuo Komai to the acceleration of the hepatic functions.

The physiology of moxibustion has been much studied in Japan by Katsusuke Serizawa, Yamashita, Tokieda, Hara Takino, Harada, Kashida, Goto, Tanisa, Kinoshita, etc. According to these writers, moxibustion provokes polynucleosis in the blood, an increase of diapedesis and phagocytary power, raising the rate of sedimentation of the red corpuscles. It increases the proportion of glucose and bicarbonate of soda, and it affects the potassium and calcium content. It is thought to cause the appearance in the system of a substance related to histamine, called histotoxin, which has been shown to be toni-cardiac, tending to raise the proportion of haemoglobin and antallergic.[6] The microtraumatism caused by the moxa or the needle also has an effect upon the autonomic nervous system.[7]

A great deal of clinical and experimental research on the subject of acupuncture has taken place since the Second World War. Morita has constructed an apparatus which will record the twelve radial pulses by the graphic method. Yoshio Manaka has invented a dermatometer (skin tester) for locating acupunctures points by means of a galvano-potentiometer with three scales.

At the present time there are in Japan thirty thousand practitioners in acupuncture or moxibustion, qualified after a three-year course of higher education. About 2,500 people enter each year for the diploma examination which is supervised by the State. The three great societies of acupuncture practitioners are the *Nihon Shinkyu Shikai* (10,000 members), the *Nihon Shinkyu Massage Shikai Renmei* (10,000 members) and the *Nihon Shinkyu Gakkai* (2,000 members).

Indian Medicine

The great works (*Samhitâ*) which make up the corpus of Ayur-Vedic medicine, coming from the oral tradition which saw the birth of the *Brahmana* and the *Upanisad*, were formed over a period of a thousand years which began with the fifth century BC.

These works, which have as yet no precise chronology, were founded (like the other four sciences of India) on the theories of the breath, of the humours and of the constituent elements of the microcosm and the macrocosm. This was a very different conception from the Chinese hypotheses, referring only to the two principles and eight trigrams to account for the perpetual transformation of things, whether in the physical or the moral world. Tsou Yen (*c.* 305–240 BC) tried to amalgamate ideas of Chinese origin with new Western notions which he probably received from

Indian travellers. In so doing he introduced an important innovation, that of the five elements (*wu-hjng*) and their gyration, and of the reciprocal destruction and genesis of these five natural agents (*Hou Wai-lu*). By analogy with the dialectic adopted in the Middle and Near East, systems of physics, medicine and alchemy were possible, and it was in fact at this period that alchemy made its appearance as a quasi-science in China. One of its component ideas was that of acquiring immortality by material means with or without the addition of religious practices. Traces of the Indo-European immortality potions can be seen here: the Iranian *haoma* (described in the *Avesta*) and the Indo-Aryan *soma* (described in the *Rig-Veda*). For centuries Taoists and alchemists were to seek the elixir of life in plants and pills, and also in breathing, dietetic and sexual techniques.

The golden age of Ayur-Vedic medicine coincides with Buddhism's period of ephemeral glory in India (327 BC–AD 750) and the great period of continental and maritime expansion which carried India's influence abroad. Among the Buddha's attendants there featured two doctors, Kasparja and Jivaka, the last of whom later became a patron of Tibetan medicine to whom tradition ascribes extraordinary operations carried out under anaesthesia by Indian hemp (laparotomy, thoracotomy and cranial trepanation). The last mentioned, an operation known as early as the Palaeolithic era, caused a great repercussion throughout Asia. The two surgeons of Chinese antiquity, Pien Ts'io (*c*. 400 BC) and Hua T'o (*c*. AD 136/141–208) are credited with wonderful treatments which are probably Chinese versions of an Indian technique, the actual origin of which has passed into legend. What is certain is that Ayur-Vedic surgery was the most remarkable in Eurasian antiquity. Although its extensive instrumental stock was partially reproduced in Tibetan works, it never roused the interest of the Chinese who, in this respect, borrowed nothing from India.

The golden age of Chinese Buddhism was from the fourth to the tenth century, during which time courageous pilgrim-monks established links in both directions between China and India. An account by Cheng Wen-ming (634–713), whose monastic name was I-tsing, has preserved their names from the initial journey made by Fa-Hien (399–414), including the most famous pilgrimage of all, that of Hiuan Tsang (629–45), to the last, which took place c.695, at the time when the Moslem barrier was about to close the Silk Road.

I-tsing returned from his pilgrimage to the holy places of Buddhism (671–95) with the Chinese translation of an Indian medical work. By referring to Nâgârjuna, the author of two alchemistic manuscripts, the *Kacchaputa* and the *Rasaratnâkara* and the collection of the 'Hundred Formulae' (*Yogacataka*), which was printed in Ceylon as late as 1898, he established that whereas the Chinese had an understanding of Indian therapeutics, the Indians took no account in their symptomatology either of the inspection of the tongue or of sphygmology (Reddy, 1938–42).

It is true that the classic collections (*Samhitâ*) of Bhela, Sucruta and Garaka made no mention of the examination of the pulse, which did not appear in Ayur-Vedic medicine until Bhaisajayagura (728–86). Towards the end of the Middle Ages and at the beginning of the modern period, sphygmology was the subject of works such as Kanada's *Nadivijnana*. It then became possible to make firmer diagnoses of illnesses caused by each of the three morbid principles (*dosa:* wind, phlegm and bile) or by their combination (*sannipata*).

Sphygmology was in the first place borrowed by Ayur-Vedic medicine from China; but Galenic theories, arriving via the Irano-Arab intermediary, also accumulated around this Chinese nucleus in addition probably to the personal observations of Indian doctors.

It will cause no surprise to see the mention of works before the time of Johann Gensfleisch or Gutenberg (c.1400–68). A fully detailed account of the discovery of printing in China has been written by Professor Liou Chuo-chiun (1958) in three versions: (a) Chinese (*Chung-kuo-shu ti ku-shih*), (b) English (*Story of the Chinese Book*), (c) Russian (*Rasskaz o kitaiskoi knige*). The oldest printed book in the world is the *Diamond Soûtra* (868). Indian admirers of Chinese civilisation were responsible for spreading the knowledge of printing techniques.

Buddhism has always attached great importance to 'bringing relief to any pain suffered by any animate being, human or animal'. It was therefore understandable that archaeologists should find a considerable number of medical texts by the side of canonical documents. About 527 Bodidharma, whose Chinese name was Ta-mo, developed a doctrine similar to that of *mens sana in corpore sano*. This was the *dhyâna* (*ch'an* in Chinese) which aimed to keep monks, wearied by their day of prayer, as physically fit as possible. It taught them the principles of efficient self-defence by boxing and other exercises which in Japan became *ju-jitsu* and *karate*.

Dhyâna is simply a Buddhist form of *yoga* which with varying modifications found its way into all the religions and philosophies of India. In this autonomous, voluntary discipline of human behaviour (Masson-Oursel) breathing exercises are of great importance. In this respect there are remarkable similarities in Taoist gymnastics (*nei-kung*): although it is not possible to assert that the Taoists owe the whole of their science to the *yogin*, both are founded on the principle of the control (*hing-ch'i*) and holding of the breath (*pi-ch'i*). (p. 226.)

Buddhism preached a theory of four elements, which probably owed something to Greek influence. It set the number of known diseases at 404, each element being responsible for 101 diseases. Lack of harmony among the elements was the cause of illness. Except during the T'ang period the Chinese classical school rarely resorted to this etiology, but at that time it was found necessary to bring the Chinese and Indian pathogenic systems into agreement. We have shown elsewhere that this attempt at compromise was particularly noteworthy in the case of Sun Szu-miao (581–682), whose memory was celebrated with great ceremony by the Chinese Academy of Medicine (Peking, 1962). Buddhist influence continued in a system of medical assistance which included hospitals, leper wards and dispensaries in the larger monasteries, and which were supported by income from 'compassion fields'. This system was

92

secularised towards the middle of the ninth century.[8] In this way
Chinese medicine acquired ethical principles of the highest order.

Of the 779 plants described in the *Pen-ts'ao chang-mu*, 211 are
common to India and China.[9] Among Chinese borrowings from
India we may note: Indian hemp (*Cannabis sativa*), datura,
chaulmoogra, sandalwood, cardamom from Malabar, Indian
camphor, cinnamon from Ceylon, long pepper, cane-sugar, etc.
Chaulmoogra is obtained from the oleaginous seeds of various
trees belonging to the family *Flacourtiaceae*, brought into European
medicine by Hobson in 1854.

India also exported works on magic and its exorcism, as in the
case of the *Kumaratantra* by Ravana, a book on antidemoniacal
medicine written in Sanskrit. There were Tibetan, Chinese, Cam-
bodian and Arab works of a similar nature (J. Filliozat, *Cahiers
Soc. As.* 1937).

Irano-Arab Medicine

Chang Ch'ien made the first break-through to the Middle East by
visiting Ferghana (*Ta-yuan*) and pointing out to the Emperor
Wu Ti (140–87 BC) the route to India, Iran and the Caspian Sea,
i.e. the Silk Road, along which Chinese and Moslems met in the
eighth century. Arab medicine is in fact neither Moslem nor the
exclusive work of the Arabs, but simply the medicine of the Arabic
language, which from the ninth to the fourteenth century had
become the international medium of Eurasian science. In Asia as
a whole it was in competition with Persian which was for a long
time the lingua franca of the Silk Road.

Well before the hegira, the pomegranate (*Punica granatum*),
which the Romans had brought back from Carthage, arrived in
China by way of Kabul (126 BC). Preceded by the radish, lucerne
(*mu-su*, 138–26 BC) or purple medic (*Medicago sativa*), the *alfalfa* of
Irano-Arabs and Americans, was the food of the famous horses of
Ferghana. It was known to the Chinese and the Greeks and came
into the empire with them.

In the third century maritime connections were established between the Persian Gulf and Canton and brought flax, hemp, walnuts, bamboos and saffron to the Far East.

The first embassy from the Commander of the Faithful (*emir al-mumenin*) arrived in China in 651 and was received by the T'ang Emperor Kao-tsung. Between 651 and 798 another thirty Arab (*Ta-shih*, Cantonese: *Tai-shik* or *Tadjik*) embassies crossed Central Asia, while Canton continued to be a main terminus for Arab maritime trade. The transfer of the Imperial capital to Hangchow under the Southern Sung dynasty favoured the development of trade by sea with a considerable exchange between the Far East, the Indian Archipelago, India and Africa. The *Hai-yo pen-ts'ao* ('Materia Medica Maritima') compiled by Li Siun during the reign of Su-tsung (756–62) introduced drugs imported from India and the Near East. The *Hu pen-ts'ao* was a book on *Hu* (probably Sogdian and Iranian) remedies. Tuan Ch'eng-shih (*c*.800) in his *You-yang tsa-tsu*, Chou Chiu-fei (*Ling-wai tai-ta*, 1178) and Chao Ju-kua in his description of foreign countries (*Chu-fan-chih*, 1225) described the products of the Persian (*po-szu*) *materia medica*. Chao Ju-kua, an inspector of trade at Ts'iuan-chou (Fukien), unfortunately confused products of Iranian origin with those from southern India (Malabar Coast), Cambodia and the Indian Archipelago. He identified from 385 to 999 of them according to the Annals of the Wei (385–556), Sui (589–617) and Sung (960–1279) dynasties. His work, which in the fifteenth century was included in the *Yung-lo ta-tien* encyclopedia, has been translated by Hirth and Rockhill. Hsia Nai made a careful study of the products of the countries now known as Kenya and Tanganyika, and of *Pi-p'a-lo* (Berbera in Somalia), *Ts'eng-pa* (Zanzibar) and *Ch'un-lun-ts'eng-chi* (Madagascar ?). He acquainted the Chinese with north Africa (*Wu-zu-li* or *Misor*), Alexandria (*Ho-chen-t'o*) and Maghreb (*Mu-lan-p'i*). These details are confirmed by archaeological discoveries which have restored Chinese coins and porcelain in Tanganyika, Zanzibar and Zimbabwe (Rhodesia). From these regions the Chinese learnt of the existence of foreign animals: the giraffe (*tsula*), the zebra and the 'camel-crane' (ostrich). Of greater interest was the acquisition of new medicines: olibanum, dragon's blood, ambergris, myrrh (from the Arabic *murr*; Chinese: *moyo*), fenugreek (Arabic *hulba*; Chinese *huluba*), opium (Arabic *afiun*; Chinese *afujong*), theriac (Arabic *tiryaq*; Chinese *ti-yih-chia*). The last mentioned was presented to the Imperial Court by a Byzantine embassy.

It may be assumed that the Arabs had a reciprocal knowledge of Chinese medicine. Laufer has compared the *Book on the Establishing of Remedies and their Properties* by Abu Mansur Muwaffaq (970) with various similar Chinese works, particularly the *Pen-ts'ao kang-mu*. Laufer's list of Chinese borrowings from Persia is: lucerne, grapes, sesame, flax, onions, shallots, peas, soya, saffron, jasmine, henna, manna, asafoetida, gall-nut, indigo, pepper, sugar, myrobolan, cumin, basil, pistachio, narcissus, date-palm, spinach, lettuce, castor oil, almonds, locust-beans, water-melon, fenugreek, *nux vomica*, carrots, styrax, myrrh, benjamin, pomegranates, coriander, walnuts, opium, etc.

Conversely, products imported to Persia from China were: bamboo, silk, peaches, apricots, cinnamon, *Cinnamomum cassia*, *Coptis teeta*, rhubarb, China rose, kaolin, tutenag, pewter and China root (Chinese sarsaparilla).

Rhazes (864–925) mentions in his alchemy a Chinese metal (*Kharsini*) which has never been accurately identified. His ethical conceptions and his description of smallpox might possibly be traceable to Far Eastern origins, since the first description of the disease was (as noted already) by Ko Hung (*c.* 281–340). It has also been assumed (by Needham) that he was visited by a Chinese scholar in Baghdad but we have no proof of this. Observations of a similar nature could be made of Avicenna (980–1037). Certain passages of the *Pen-ts'ao chang-mu* ('Classification of Medicinal Insects and Soils') and of his *Canon of Medicine* have been shown to have a close resemblance. Gruner has also noted parallels between the Arab and Chinese sphygmologies, but all this is at present a matter of surmise. After the fall of the Sung dynasty,

Chinese–Moslem relations became extremely important.

During this period, which was the time of Marco Polo (1271–95), the foreign Yüan dynasty (1280–1368) with Kublai Khan (1257–94) was reigning over China, while another Mongol, Hulagu (1256–65) had become the ruler of Iran. In his third journey Marco Polo (who never went to Africa) mentioned Sokotra, Madagascar, Zanzibar and Ethiopia, probably as a result of Chinese references. But he could possibly have known the accounts of Suleiman (ninth century), the first merchant to write on China, and of Ali el Masudi (tenth century). In 1307 he landed in the Persian Gulf, a region already long frequented by Chinese vessels. A little later Ibn Batuta (1304–77) established a link between Morocco and Hangchow and brought knowledge of the Far East to north Africa. Whatever the case, with foreign practitioners Chinese medicine received Arab lapidaries, Indian chaulmoogra, alcohol, opium and mandragora. Irano-Arabian medicine received Chinese texts and rhubarb. Tabriz was the main link for these Chinese, Iranian and Mongol encounters promoted by the *Pax Mongolica*. The prime mover was Rashid al-Din (*c*. 1247–1318), also called Rashid al-Din Tabib, who was successively physician and prime minister to Mahmud Ghazan Khan (1295–1304), the grandson of Hulagu, and to the Il-Khan Uljai-tu (1304–17) whose kingdoms stretched from the Oxus to the Euphrates. He built hospitals at Hamadan (his birth-place and that of Avicenna), Shiraz and Tabriz where Indian, Syrian, Iranian and Chinese doctors worked together. The name of one, Siyuse (?), has been preserved, and a disputation between a Byzantine doctor and Rashid al-Din has been recorded. Rashid al-Din brought in Chinese medicines and books and took advantage of his position as the prime minister of a Mongol prince to compile a historical encyclopedia which embraced almost all the peoples of Eurasia, from the Central Empire to 'frankish' Christendom. He used this store of reference to compose an encyclopedia in Persian: *The Il-Khan's treasury of the Sciences of Cathay* (1313), one copy of which is to be found in St Sophia's Library at Istanbul (ms. no. 3596). This work, under its Turkish title *Tanksuknamei*

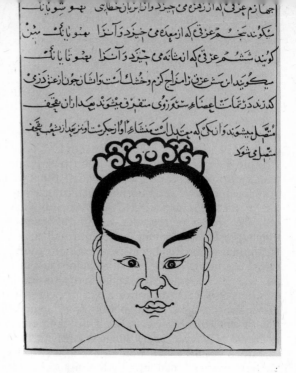

Il-han der fünuru ulúmu hatai mukaddimesi, has been the subject of study by Adnan and Professor Süheyl Unver. It consists of four volumes, translated into Persian from a text in *Hataki* (Chinese Turkestan). The manuscript's first page is decorated with an illumination, and bears the seal of Mahmud I and its catalogue number (3596) in St Sophia's Library. The first and most important volume begins with an introduction of seventy pages written by Rashid al-Din himself. It is illustrated with numerous figures and diagrams of Chinese authorship with captions in Irano-Arabic and is a translation of the *Mo-ching* by Wang Shu-ho. A second volume considers the treatment of affections of the circulatory system by cauteries and moxas. The third volume is in two parts which contain dialogues between rulers and their ministers, a classification of ancient books, the therapeutic effects of certain medicines demonstrated in two separate chapters, and finally the methods used in the treatment of illnesses by *Hataki* doctors before they acquired knowledge of Greek medicine. The fourth volume is

A folio from the great scientific encyclopedia
(*The Il-Khan's Treasury of the Sciences of Cathay*)
compiled by Rashid al-Din. The four Persian
volumes are based on a text from Chinese Turkestan.
During the *Pax Mongolica* considerable medical
interchange took place.

devoted to *Hataki* medical doctrine and its classification of diseases. The facing illustration shows a page from this work.

Irano-Turko-Arab medicine made very extensive use of actual cauteries. Igneous cauterisation, using points which are sometimes very localised and at a considerable distance from the lesions, was one of the methods favoured by Sabundjuoglu Shereffetin (1404–68), the author of the oldest Turkish book on surgery.[10] It is difficult to say whether a clear Chinese influence can be seen in this technique, since Rashid al-Din seems to have been much more interested in the doctrine of the pulse than in moxibustion. This last was one of the most popular forms of treatment in Egypt and was first referred to in Europe by Prospero Alpini (1553–1617), a Venetian who spent a long period as a doctor in Egypt. In his *De Plantis Aegyptii*, 1591, in which coffee is first mentioned, and later in his *De Medicinae Aegyptorum*, he described cauteries with a base of carded cotton which were in use in Cairo. He made no use of the term *moxa* (coined later by Kaempfer) but gave them the name *ustio* or *adustio* (therapeutic burn). After him Johann Vesling (1610–49), a professor at Pavia, visited Egypt and praised its method of cauterisation. Dominique Larrey was the last great European surgeon to mention it. If the Egyptian cotton moxa and the Chinese mugwort moxa are not two separate discoveries, but have instead a common origin to be found either in Egypt or in China, it is possible that the Mongols who arrived in the Nile delta towards 1263–96 (with ten thousand tents) were the disseminators of this technique, as of other techniques which came from Central Asia (paper and printing). An intermediary between Egypt and Asia could have been Iran. There are in fact allusions to acupuncture and moxas in the Denkart. It was probably the Moslem world which acquainted China with maize or Indian corn, observed at the end of the sixteenth century by T'ien I-heng (1573), Shen Mou-kuan (1581), Wang She-mu (1587), and Li Shih-chen (1590) who gave the first illustrations of it. The Moslems of Spain and north Africa could have made it known at Mecca, and from there it could have reached the Far East either over land through

A Sino-Vietnamese pharmacy. Note
the two instruments typical of
the dispensary, the herb-chopper
worked by the man and the bronze
vessel (*thuyen*) operated by
the woman's feet.

Central Asia or by the maritime route via India. During the Ming
period Cheng-ho (1371–1435), a famous Moslem of Yünnan
(whose father and grandfather had made the pilgrimage to Mecca)
made seven voyages in the Indian Ocean between 1405 and 1433.
These brought him in the north to the Red Sea and in the south to
Sokotra, Cape Guardafui, Hafun, Mogadiscio, Brava, the mouth
of the River Futa, Malindi and Mombasa. Cheng-Ho's collabora-
tors, Ma-Huan, Fei-Sin and Chung-chen left valuable accounts of
their voyages: *Ying-yai-sheng-lan* ('Description of Lands and Seas'),
Sing-ch'aisheng-lan ('Description of Distant Lands') and *Si-yang
fan-kuo chih* ('Report on the Foreign Countries beyond the Eastern
Ocean'). They show that, eighty years before the arrival of the
Portuguese, Afro-Asian links were firmly established and with them
significant exchanges in *materia medica* between China, India and
the Arab world.

The barrier eventually placed between India and Africa by the
Portuguese was not always effective. In the sixteenth century
'China root' (*radix Chinae*) had acquired such a reputation in the
treatment of syphilis that Vesalius himself devoted a letter to the
subject. From China it arrived in Goa, and from there it was sent
both to Europe and to the Moslem countries as far as Morocco
under the Persian name *cub i Cini* (China wood) and the Arabic
names of *gubsini*, *subsini* and *djoutchi*.[11]

Vietnamese Medicine

The tropic of Cancer, passing through Dong Van (to the north-
east of Ha Giang), leaves below it the greater part of Vietnam
whose climate, ethnic stock, fauna and flora are very different from
their Chinese counterparts. Essentially one might say that Vietnamese doctors are obliged to import many Chinese medicinal
plants (*thuôc bac*), but the Chinese 'uncle' cannot do without
certain much sought-after tropical species (*thuôc nam*) which he
has had to buy from his 'nephews' in the south. Roughly speaking
these amount to a score of zingiberaceous plants (galingale,

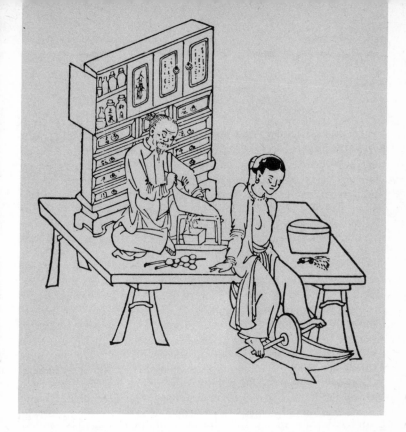

amomum, ginger, betony, sweet cyperus, quisqualis, etc.) and four important plants: cassia (*nyuc quê*), cardamom (*bach dâu khâu*), the famous eagle wood which does not grow north of the 14th parallel (*trâm huong*) and the aloe (*lô hoi*). There is a Chinese proverb which caustically asserts that the Vietnamese is dying under a heap of drugs, and there is no better way of implying that he fails to obtain the best advantage from the many medicinal plants growing in his country. It was appropriately with a herbal, by *Phan-Phu-Tiên* (*Ban-thao tu-vât toan-yêu*, 1429), that Vietnamese medical literature began. Nguyên Thuc was the author of a book on hygiene (*Bao-anh luong-phuong*, fifteenth century) recast by the order of King Lê Hi-tông as a 'Précis on the Preserving of Life and the Prolonging of Old Age' (*Bao-sinh duyên-tho toan-yêu*, 1676). But the first Sino-Vietnamese to show proof of originality was a scholar-bonze who lived for a long time in China. His name Tuê-tinh, is not a patronymic but a monastic name which may have been borne by several bonzes in succession from the tenth to the seventeenth century. The man we are concerned with may have lived at the beginning of the fifteenth century under the name of *Hông Nghia*. He was a connoisseur of the *Pen-ts'ao* (Vietnamese: *Ban-thao*) and a specialist in drugs. He left one manuscript, the original of which has been lost, but which was reproduced by wood-engravings in 1717, 1726 and 1762 with the titles *Hông Nghia giac-ti y-thu* (Hông Nghia's book of medicine for the instruction of the people) and *Nam-duoc thân-hiêu* ('Wonderful Efficacy of the Remedies of the South'). The work is written in classical Chinese characters with Vietnamese demotic characters (*chu-nôm*) to designate the local flora and is interspersed with passages of rhythmic prose (*phu*). Six hundred and fifty remedies from the three realms of nature are studied in this way. They were chosen, not from the stock of Chinese *Pen-ts'ao* which would not have been suitable 'for the people south of the marches', but from a fauna and flora perfectly adapted to the Vietnamese temperament. Tuê-tinh is reminiscent of the German Renaissance doctors who aimed to cure their patients by substituting herbs which grew in central or northern Europe for the medicinal plants of the Mediterranean and Arab regions. At an early date he was regarded as the patron of Vietnamese doctors.[12]

The eighteenth century produced several important doctors. Nguyén Nho and Ngo-van-Tinh compiled a collection of herbs to which they added an extract from the inevitable *Pen-ts'ao chang-mu* ('General Compendium of Materia Medica') by Li Shih-chen, put into Vietnamese with the title *Ban-thao cuong-muc*. Another therapeutist, Nguyen cong Triên, listed three hundred Sino-Vietnamese remedies in his *Thuc vat tiep luc* (1752). Nguyen gia Phan studied epidemic diseases in his *Lieu dich phuong phap* (1788). Ngo-van-Tinh (a doctor in 1763) with his *Van phuong tap nghiem* and Nguyên-Thê-lich (*Thai dien dony y*, 1777 and *Tien nhu Khoa*, c.1782) were gynaecologists. Nguyen-Thê-Lich (*Thai tien dien duong*, 1771) has left a manual of pediatrics. All were eclipsed by the great figure of Lê-huu-Chân (1720 – later than 1786) whose pseudonym, Lan Ong, means 'the old man with time on his hands'. He was steeped in Chinese culture and was successful in the three examinations for literary studies. After service as a soldier he fell seriously ill and then retired to the country to devote himself to divination. He subsequently spent ten years studying the Chinese medical classics and afterwards, in accordance with the best Confucian tradition, opened a literary, philosophical and medical school in his cottage *Huong-son* ('the scented mountain') near Ha-tinh, where he wrote a number of books. His encyclopedia is in six books and twenty-six chapters. The first edition, dating from 1770, must have been in manuscript, but there were wood-engravings in the editions of 1866 and 1879–85.[13]

Lan Ong's sources are exclusively Chinese. He seems particularly to have used the classic on internal medicine (*Nei-ching*), Chang Chung-ching's 'Ailments Attributable to Cold' (*Shang-han-lun*), the general compendium of *materia medica* (*Pen-ts'ao chang-mu*) and authors of the Ts'ing period: Yu Chang and Feng Ch'ao-chang. There can be no doubt that he admired them, but without any sacrifice either of his originality or his individuality. He knew that the medical geography of tropical Vietnam was not that of temperate China, and he wished to work out a therapeutic method adapted to his national soil rather than borrowed from abroad. In this respect he followed the lead of Tuê-tinh, but he outstripped him through his extensive knowledge of medical thought and clinical practice, through his talent as a writer and the originality with which he corrected the classical theories in the light of his own experience 'in order to draw new conceptions from them' (*Study on the Medical Source of the Sea*, 1782). Elsewhere he recommends his pupils to 'strive to get to the bottom of things and never to follow word for word the old methods of treatment when applying them to patients whose resistance is lowered. In such a case failure is certain'. (*Simple Therapeutics for Ailments Attributable to External Causes*.) He added: 'Medicine is very complicated. It can assume thousands of aspects and yet it has one sole principle which is founded on reason' (*The Jade Precepts*).

The Emperor Gia-Long, founder of the Nguyên dynasty (1802–20), had a brilliant reign. In legislation, protocol and literature the influence of Peking remained supreme and the prescriptions drawn up for the sick ruler followed the complicated regulations of Chinese therapeutics. An administration was set up (1805–14) and the teaching of medicine was organised in the capital, Hué.

There had long been in existence a corporation for doctors who worshipped their protecting spirits at certain anniversaries in buildings called temples although they had no religious character. Just as throughout Vietnam there were temples of literature (*Van miêu*) in which scholars paid their respects to Confucius, so there were temples of medicine (*Y miêu*). At a very early date Tuê-tinh was venerated in the pagoda of Hong Van. A building of this nature was still in existence at Hanoi in 1954. The main altar consisted of three central slabs consecrated to the three legendary emperors: Fu Hsi (in the centre), Shen Nung (on the right) and Huang Ti (on the left). The lateral slabs, contrary to Chinese custom, were those of the two greatest Vietnamese doctors, Tuê-tinh on the right and Lan Ong on the left. Two panels surmounted the lateral altars. The panel over the right-hand altar stated it to be that of eminent Sino-Vietnamese doctors of past centuries, called 'the western congregation', and the panel over the left-hand altar dedicated it to doctors, saints and sages of earlier periods, forming 'the eastern congregation'.

The society of North-Vietnamese doctors and pharmacists celebrated three annual feasts in this temple, one to the honour of Lan Ong, one to the Emperor Shen Nung and a third to commemorate the society's foundation (*Tong-chi Bac Viêt*).[14] Nguyen Dich (*Van Khê y ly yêu luc*, 1885) was one of the first authors to reveal a Western influence, in particular on the subject of anatomy.

Public interest in medical themes gave rise to popularisations, the best of which are those written by Nguyên Dinh Chiêu (1822–65), who became a doctor in 1843. He was the author of a 'dialogue

A medical examination at the court of Hue in the nineteenth century. Western medicine began to take root in Vietnam from the second half of the century, but for more than fifty years was opposed by traditionalists as unsuited to the country. Today it coexists alongside Sino-Vietnamese medicine and indigenous herbal remedies.

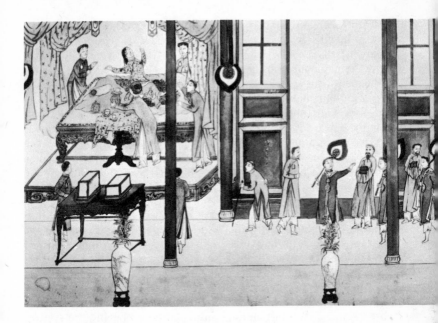

between a fisherman and a woodcutter on the art of medicine' in six- and eight-character Chinese verse written in demotic Vietnamese (*chu nôm*). Part of his famous poem *Luc van tiên* is also on the subject of medicine.

Although Sino-Vietnamese medicine suffered from a large number of charlatans who had no knowledge of botany or of Chinese characters, nevertheless its high ethical code and its efficiency were extolled by Père de Rhodes (1591–1660), whose opinion was confirmed by Padre Cristoforo Borri (seventeenth century). Padre João de Loureiro (1715–94) and Monsignor Taberd (1794–1840).[15]

From about 1860 Vietnam was invaded by Western medicine, which had for some time gained a foothold in the court at Hué but had not been propagated on a national scale. The reactions provoked by this invasion, and the counter-attack from traditional medicine, have been studied by Dr Le-Quang-Trinh (1911), the first Vietnamese to obtain the state doctorate in medicine, and his colleagues Buu Hiêp (1936), Pham Huy-Dan (1949), Le Van-Trien (1952), Pham Phu-Kha (1952) and Pham Trong-Luong (1952).

Some Vietnamese have been fanatical admirers of Western medicine, regarding radiography, capable of seeing all and knowing all, as the supreme diagnostic medium. Similarly they have considered European medicines to be capable of curing everything. But the sceptical and the opponents of Western medicine were of greater number. For them its over-simple sphygmology inspired no confidence as a means of diagnosis and prognosis, while European dietetics were a poor affair compared with the part played in traditional practice by the diet with its permitted foods and taboos. Certain therapeutic methods frightened them. The application of ice could only be dangerous in *yin* diseases. There were contra-indications for anthelmintics as being too effective, since for a healthy child the presence of a few parasites was proof of his fitness. Taking even the smallest sample of blood destroyed 'breaths' and vital principles, consequently weakening the system. Electric treatments were harmful and medicinal injections dangerous for infants. Furthermore surgery, the favourite form of European therapeutics, did not always bring about a cure, and when it did this was often at the price of bodily mutilation, forbidden by filial piety which required that a child should die in the condition it was in at birth.

From a general point of view, since medicines were adapted to a given country and population, Western medicines were not considered suitable for the Vietnamese. They over-heated; their action was rapid and short-lived; they caused male sterility, etc. In spite of this, Western medicine began to expand considerably in Vietnam after 1914. Since 1936, Doctors of Medicine, trained on the spot and continuing with courses of further study abroad, were gradually able to take over all the services required by a modern

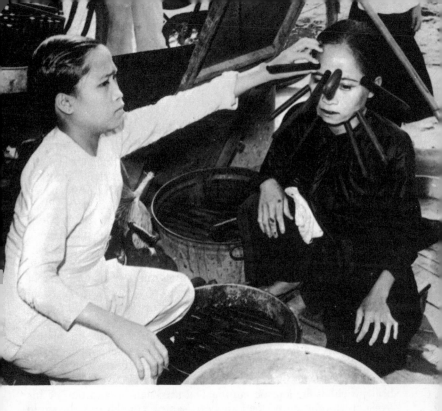

country. Yet traditional medicine nevertheless went on living at its own slow pace. In the provinces the European pharmacy, the Sino-Vietnamese town pharmacy (importing 75 per cent of its drugs from China) and the Vietnamese village dispensary (selling almost exclusively local products) continued to exist together. They fulfilled their social function, which was to ensure for everyone, from the richest to the poorest, from the most Westernised to the least developed, the ability to be cared for by one of the country's three medical systems. The medical association of the Vietnam Centre (*Trung-Ky Y-hoc-hôi*) fostered a public understanding of medicinal plants, and for a long time in rural areas entropion was still being treated in accordance with a surgical procedure dating from the Sung dynasty: the compression of the upper eyelid in a bamboo clip. After decolonisation traditional medicine developed along the lines indicated at the start of this chapter.

The Medicine of Central Asia

The Silk Road brought China into early contact with the Turko-Mongol nomads and the settled states of Khotan (*Yu-t'ien*), Turfan (*Kao-ch'ang*), Kutch (*Kien-tzu*) and Tibet. Fu Chien founded a Tibetan dynasty which ruled northern China with an enlightened and humane administration. He tried to conquer the rest of the Chinese world but was defeated on the Fei, a river in the province of Ngan-huei, in 383.[16]

At a later date, Indo-Iranian ideas and Chinese medical thought were exchanged by caravans and missionaries of the various religions.

Christian heresies such as Nestorianism (seventh to tenth centuries), Mazdaism and Manichaeism (ninth to thirteenth centuries) had great cultural significance until the Mongol period.

According to Toynbee, Nestorianism forms the chrysalis of the Christian civilisation of the Far East, a civilisation which, though abortive, was the response to conditions resulting from the disintegration of Hellenistic culture and the birth of a culture of the West. It developed in the basin of the Oxus and Iaxartes only to be extinguished with the annexation of that area by the Arabs (737–41). After a complete break of nine centuries with the Syrian world it gave Central Asia a life of its own, thanks (in the early stages) to the large number of Greek colonisers and to its special nature as a region lying on the great commercial routes. This culture was responsible for the spread of the Aramaic alphabet from Egypt to the satrapies of north-west India (Indo-Aramaic script: *kharosthi*) and to North and Central Asia (*Uigur*). It may have contributed to the dispersal of astronomical, astrological and alchemist ideas as also of acupuncture, moxas and the doctrine of the pulse.

Tibet and Mongolia were the two sectors within the immense field of influence of the Tibetan church and its medicine. We shall take no account of pre-Buddhist medicine, related to the popular medicine of north-west China. We shall consider only the

Below and overleaf Tibetan anatomical charts. For all its isolation Tibet borrowed widely from abroad, calling on Sanskrit, Pali and Chinese works for its medical sources

107

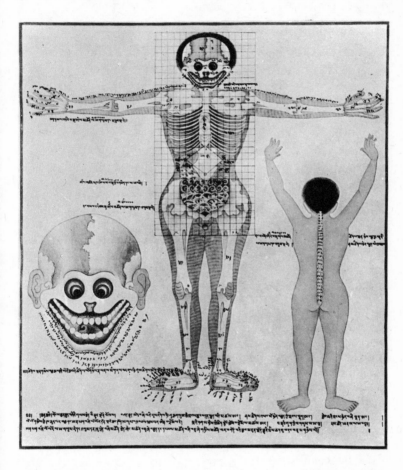

Buddhist period, bearing in mind that medicine always played a major part in a country which was often called the 'land of medicinal plants' and the country of medicine. Towards the seventh century Tibetan civilisation was overtaken by that of India, brought

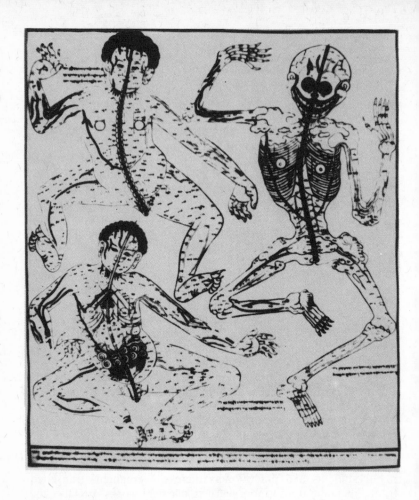

(*c.*650) by Buddhist missionaries. From the seventh to the ninth century the Mongols were converted to Buddhism and to the medicine of Tibet. Thus Mongol medicine is a replica of Tibetan, with borrowings from the medicine of China and the West.[17] Tibeto-Mongolian medicine presents two aspects: popular and scientific. In popular medicine Shamanism played a great part, being of course one of the oldest institutions of Central Asia. It held out against Buddhism and found its way into lamaism in the form of exorcism, spells, tantrist rites and bloody sacrifices. The most recognisable traces of Shamanism were to be found in the northern Buriat Mongols, grouped around Lake Baikal.[18]

Many lamas who were experts in magic and initiated into tantrism (*sgappa*) were partial shamans. They made healing and protective talismans for use both externally (formulas or magic shapes) and internally (pellets of barley flour containing amulets). Many diseases were treated magically by the intervention of Bodhisattvas or of doctor-Buddhas who neutralised the malignant influences of evil spirits. The greatest of the Bodhisattvas after Avalokitesvara was Mandjusri.

The Mongols were experienced healers and some of their practices passed over into Europe by way of Russia (Karell's milk diet). At the end of the nineteenth century a Buriat, Shamsaran, a godson of Alexander III, worked up for himself a fine practice of female clients at St Petersburg. The scientific medicine of Tibet had a monastic following and nearly all the lamaist monasteries of any size had centres for medical studies with anatomo-physiological charts, libraries and dispensaries. Under the sign of Jivaka, Buddha's contemporary and companion, they gave instruction in medical theory and practice.

Mongol medicine was also taught in religious schools exclusively reserved for lamas. The studies lasted three years and could only be begun after the student had gone through a course of theology. Urga was the main centre.

For students and practitioners there were manuals translated from Tibetan and also more learned, classical works. In Tibet the teaching was based on Tibetan translations of Sanskrit, Pali or Chinese (and perhaps Iranian) texts and on a national tradition largely derived from Sanskrit medical works. The oldest of all was the *Rgyud-bzi*, popularly called the 'four tantra' (Four Books) or, more precisely, the *Bdud-rci-snin-po Amrtahrdaya*. This was a basic work compiled in the eighth century and reminiscent of the classic *Ayur-Veda*, 'Science of Longevity', agreeing, sometimes identically, with passages from Vâgbhata who, after Caraka and Sucruta, was the most important traditional medical author in India. He is thought (without great certainty) to have lived in the sixth century and to be the author of the *Rasarathâkara muccaya* (medical alchemy) and the *Astângasamgraha* (compendium of the eight-part science), of which there is an abridged version, the *Astângahr-dayasa-mhitâ*.

Other Sanskrit medical texts were later incorporated with the two great Buddhist encyclopedias, the *Kanjur* (or Tibetan *Tripitaka* in 108 volumes which were compiled from the seventh to the twelfth centuries) and the *Tanjur*. The *Kanjur* contains Nagayûna's *Yogctaka*; the *Tanjur* was the subject of an abstract in English by Csoma de Körös as early as 1835. Pozdneev (1908) produced an incomplete version based on a Mongol text and Filliozat has translated the chapter on the foundations of health and disease into French (1954). Palmyr Ulderic Alexis Cordier (1871–1914) made a study of the medical works included in the *Tanjur* (Peking red edition) and an index of the *Kanjur* was compiled by L. Feer (1830–1902).

The Pali or Chinese pathological or anatomical texts were to be found in the so-called *gsum'bum* works or the one hundred thousand words (Collection of Collections), which are preserved in the Peking National Library. These great collections were printed from wood-blocks in the great monasteries: Lithang, Dzogchen, Dégué, Narthang and Koum-Hboum.

The first European to visit Lhasa and Peking was Oderic de Pordenone (*c.* 1325 ?) who was also the only European to visit Tibet in the Middle Ages. He was followed by Padre Ippolito Desideri (*d.* 1733), who lived in Tibet from 1715 to 1721 and left a comprehensive study of lamaism which was not known until the end of the nineteenth century.

Père Parennin, the famous author of *Manchu Anatomy*, describes how the Emperor K'ang Hsi took pleasure in putting into competition with each other the medicines of the West, of China and of Tibet. One of his letters depicts Brother Paramino, the Court Surgeon, suffering a violent attack of colic while on the north-west frontier where he was a member of the emperor's retinue. No

Yoga exercises, from
a nineteenth-century
Tibetan work.

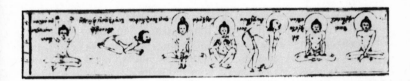

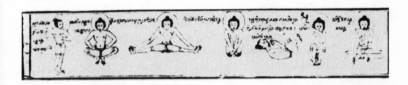

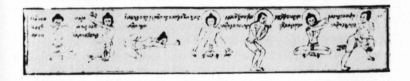

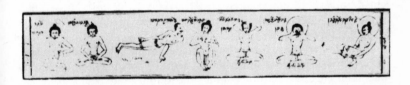

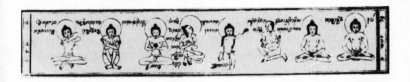

Western or Chinese doctor present in the camp was able to cure him. When he was informed, the emperor demanded advice in writing from each doctor, obtaining what amounted to a report on deficiency disease. He then summoned a Tibetan lama who cured the patient in half an hour with a voluminous suppository made on the spot with oil, wax, tow and herbal powders.

Tibetan medicine has an individual character which it derives from its thermal springs, its rich *materia medica* and its techniques. Despite the high altitude and cold climate, the Tibetan plateau holds a good number of hot springs. Over a distance of more than five miles in the region round Lac Tzegadan in the north, springs of boiling water issuing from calcium carbonate rock are connected with subterranean pockets of gas. In the mountains of Lhasa there are geysers which spurt to a height of ten feet at a temperature of 80°C. There are no fewer than three hundred species of plant and natural medicinal substance such as *Gynura pinnatifida*, rhubarb (*Rheum officinale*), angelica (*Archangelica officinalis*), fritillary (*Fritillaria roylei*), *Aweto* (caterpillar parasitised by the fungus *Cordyceps*), *Gastrodia elata*, *Codonopsis tangshen*, *Ephedra sinica*, *Scopolia japonica* and many more. *Aweto* is employed as a very rare tonic in China and more than fifty tons are produced annually. *Scopolia japonica*, famous as a medicinal plant throughout the world, grows in abundance in Himalaya, and a considerable number of Tibetan herbs are used in Western medicine as well as in the traditional medicine of China.

The Tibetan symptomatology made use of the study of the respiratory system and of uroscopy, scorned by the Chinese elders. The lamas examined the colour, the odour and the sparkle of urine with as much attention as our medieval urinomancers with their *matula*. They would beat it with a wooden spatula to discover whether it was 'mute' or 'speaking'. They could even treat a patient in his absence simply by inspecting his urine. This would involve examination of the morning, midday, evening and night urine, and account would be taken of the colour, odour, sparkle, sound and taste.

It is nevertheless true that there was evidence of foreign influence in Tibetan medicine. Medical manuscripts give the names of the *materia medica* not only in Tibetan but often translated into Chinese or Sanskrit characters, sometimes also into Uigur or Persian. This is so in the case of a herbal preserved at the *Société Asiatique* (*Ye-ces don-grub bstan-pa'i rgyal-mchan*).

Chinese influence can be clearly defined: it was shown in the use of acupuncture and moxas, in sphygmology, the inspection of the tongue and diagnosis.

The doctrine of the pulse appeared as early as the eighth century in the fundamental work of Tibeto-Mongolian medicine, the *Rgyud-bzi*, and can only be attributed to a borrowing from China. Subsequently however, as happened in the case of India, sphygmological ideas of Greek, Arab and Iranian origin could have found their way to Tibet. Wang Shu-ho and Galen probably met.

Wet cupping and bleeding are not Chinese practices. The lamas used trumpets carved from human femurs, wands made of bone and skull-caps. They showed a certain familiarity with anatomy, and in fact the anatomical charts in Tibetan works were sometimes more carefully drawn than those of the Chinese. They illustrated the five organic centres controlling the human body (*chakra*). The heart was one of these centres, sending many ducts into the trunk and limbs. There is evidence of Indian influence here.

The numerous instruments featured in Tibetan medical books constituted a more extensive stock than the Chinese. This is not surprising when we remember that Jivaka, Buddha's doctor, 'thrice king of doctors' and the great patron of Tibetan medicine, was known for his surgical exploits, and that several doctors of the royal household were thought to have studied in India. It is known that India's surgical equipment was the most extensive in the whole of Asia, and a certain number of instruments appearing in Tibetan books may simply have been reproduced as a matter of course or by tradition and not in fact used. The instruments in general use appear to have been cauteries, cupping-glasses, lancets for blood-letting and cataract needles. Among the Turko-Mongols there was a guild of army surgeons (*Jakshi*) which also appeared among the great Mongols of India (1526–1857) and which may well have existed with the Tibetans and the Mongols. Surgery was in fact prohibited to the lamas. The therapeutic use of cinnamon, benjamin and *nux vomica* and perhaps variolation can be traced to India. Variolation was known in China in the eleventh century when Wang Tan (*c*. 1023–63) had his son inoculated by a hermit living on the Tibetan border who used a method imported from India.

A final component in Tibetan medicine is the Greek tradition brought from Iran, particularly emphasised by R. A. Stein:

Indeed according to a very serious chronicle which devotes a chapter to the history of the medicine of Tibet, an Indian doctor, Vajradhvaja, a Chinese doctor, Hen-Weng Han-De, and a doctor of Khrom (Byzantium, 'Rome'?) from Tazig (Iran) called Ga-le-nos were invited to Tibet during the lifetime of the Chinese wife of Songtse Gampo (Wen-ch'eng, seventh century). Books representing the different schools of these countries were translated, but only the 'Galen from Iran', Galenos, was appointed Physician to the King or Physician in Chief (*bla-sman*) and instructed pupils 'without regard to the rank of their families'. Later, when Princess Kin-ch'eng (eighth century) renewed the translations of works on medicine from India and China, she is thought to have invited from Khrom the doctor *Bi-chi-tsan-ba-shi-la-ha*, whose name does in fact contain the Persian word for doctor. And it was again this 'Greek from Iran' rather than a Chinese or Indian who was appointed Physician to the King (*Lha-rje*), an expression explained by the chronicle as 'lord of the King' *rgyal-po'i rje*, having the prerogative of sitting in the centre of the assembly on an 'excellent carpet' and of being venerated as superior (*blar bkur-ba*) by all the rest.

3 Medicine in China and Europe

The seventeenth and eighteenth centuries

Chinoiserie Although the discovery of China was the greatest
achievement of Western explorers in the Middle Ages, it was not
until the eighteenth century that Europe acquired a knowledge of
the Chinese race and culture. François Bernier, in the *Journal des
Savants* (24 April 1684) and the *Etrennes adressées à Madame de
Sablière pour l'année* 1688, was the first to divide human races into
four groups and to take account of a yellow element. From Marco
Polo to Albuquerque there seems in fact to have been no idea of a
yellow race, and in South-East Asia the Chinese were regarded as
'white' by peoples of deeper pigmentation. When Père Couplet
presented a young Chinese to Louis xiv on 15 September 1684,
the *Mercure Galant* of that month wrote of the 'young Indian' and
his 'Indian clothes'. The youth referred to was Michel Shen
Fu-tsung who was later to work with Thomas Hyde at Oxford
(1687), where British sinological studies first began. He was followed by another of his compatriots, Arcade Huang (1679–1716),
who was brought to France by Artus de Lyonne. Huang married a
Frenchwoman and became the assistant of the king's librarian,
Fourmont. There were by now many more Chinese in Europe,
some being in the Jesuit College at Naples. In the Jesuit house in
Paris the name of Ignace Xavier Lan (1727–96) can be found
among those of several novices entering after 1750. The last to be
mentioned were the priests Aloys Kao (1733–90 ?) and Etienne
Yang (1759–98?) who we shall refer to later in connection with
Turgot and Bertin.

After the voyages of the *Amphitrite* (1698–1703), and with the
founding of the Dutch, English and French companies in the
Indies, Chinese products (tea, cloth, wall-paper, lacquer, ceramics
and ivory) poured into a Europe which went crazy over them and
incorporated them into everyday decoration. Trade in Chinese
articles had thus reached a significant level by the end of the
seventeenth century. Later the West began to find out more about
Chinese natural products (mineral, vegetable and animal) which

featured in albums preserved at the *Bibliothèque Nationale*, the *Institut de France*, the French Museum of Natural History and the *Musée de Bretagne*. Special interest was shown in technology (agriculture, weaving, horn work, the construction of canals, and dyeing).

Art was drawn into this movement with Anglo-Chinese gardens, the furniture of Thomas Chippendale, lacquer cabinets, Chinese curios, and ceramics (pottery and porcelain) inspired by Far Eastern models.

Henri Cordier (1849–1925) has described the many aspects of this infatuation whereby Chinese themes ousted the *fleur-de-lis* on cast iron fire-places, plates from the Far East were decorated in Europe with the arms of Fouquet or Madame de Pompadour, fashionable cloths, 'nankeen' (yellow cotton) and 'pekin' (silk) were to be seen along with Chinese knives, Chinese baths, Chinese shadow pictures, and 'Chinese' candied lemons. It was the period when, following the example of Sir William Chambers (1757), Le Rouge and others built 'exotic follies' and overthrew the traditional arrangement of French gardens. It was indeed on a Chinese lacquer desk (made by Jouret) that Louis XVI wrote his will in the Temple prison.

But it was not only in the material aspects of its civilisation that China became a model for Europe. Leibnitz saw in Chinese characters the pattern for a universal script, and he hailed the pre-eminence of Chinese moral philosophy which also provided Voltaire with some of his sharpest political weapons. Not all philosophers followed the example of their enthusiasm, but the physiocrats found in the thousand-year-old Chinese Empire the best confirmation of their theories.

In Quesnay's *Despotisme de la Chine* (1767) an indubitable similarity is demonstrated between the Chinese idea of cosmic order and the primacy of agriculture and the physiocratic conception of the natural, providential World Order of which the State is the guardian, not the creator (*Ex natura, jus, ordo et leges*). The idea of competitive examination (which was to acquire considerable importance as the standard means for the selection of candidates for a post) also appears to have spread by virtue of its Chinese reputation.

It was in such an atmosphere that Henri Léonard Jean-Baptiste Bertin (1719–92), Secretary of State responsible for correspondence with China and the *Compagnie des Indes*, gathered together some very important documents in his Paris house, situated at the corner of the *Boulevards* and the *Rue Neuve des Capucines*, and in his residence at Chatou. His collections and correspondence, sold in 1792 like those of so many émigrés, are at present divided between the *Bibliothèque Nationale* (*Fonds Bréquigny*, of which twenty-two volumes are devoted to China) in the *Cabinet des Estampes*, the library of the *Institut de France* and the library of the French Museum of Natural History.

Bertin, a pioneer founder of veterinary schools (in particular that at Lyons), was interested in medicine and the biological sciences and was the protector of the anatomist Fragonard. He considered it supremely important that French missionaries should live at the Imperial Court of China, with no ulterior political or commercial motive, and thus represent French culture at one of the vital points of the Far East. To this end he did not hesitate to send anything that might give pleasure to his opposite numbers in China and he particularly approved the fact that the great series of Ch'ien Lung's victories were engraved in Paris, the international centre for engraving, by Cochin.

Together with Turgot and other prominent people, he was well aware that the first French sinologists had misunderstood Chinese psychology and needed to be corrected by a number of investigations, scientifically carried out not by Europeans, but by Chinese. It was for this purpose that he brought Aloys Kao and Etienne Yang to France (from 1751 to 1764). This was not the first time that young Chinese had come to Europe to finish their clerical studies, but Turgot and Bertin were the first to give them an excellent scientific and technical training and to send them back to China in 1766 with a generous pension and princely gifts (watches,

Westerners in Chinese eyes, as seen in the
eighteenth century from 'Illustrations of the
tributaries of the Imperial Ch'ing dynasty',
attributed to Fu Heng. *Left to right*
an Englishman, a Russian, a Pole,
and an unspecified European.

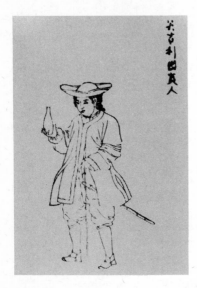
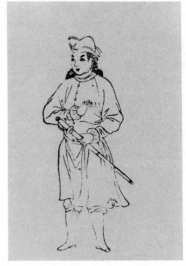

astronomical telescopes, physical apparatus, a printing press,
mirrors from St Gobain, Sèvres china, wallpapers and Beauvais
tapestries).[1]

Back in their own country, priests 'full of zeal, enlightenment
and wisdom', but foreigners in their native land, Bertin's two
protégés found themselves unable to carry out the task committed
to them, which they therefore left to the Peking missionaries.

European scholars in China The presence in Peking in the seventeenth and eighteenth centuries of a number of monks practising
medicine (Frère Bernard Rhodes, 1669–1715, Frère Jean-Joseph
da Costa, 1679–1747, Frère Etienne Rousset, 1689–1758, Frère
Emmanuel de Mattos, 1725–64, Frère Louis Bazin, 1712–74), and
Western lay physicians and surgeons (Thomas Garwin, 1716–7,
John Bell, 1720) who came with the Russian embassy, contributed
to the spread of European medicine if only through the hospital

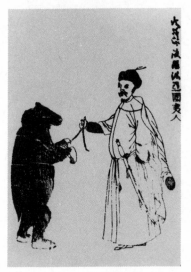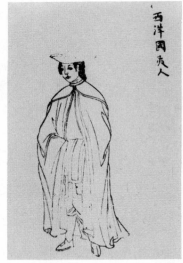

founded by Candida Siu (1607–80), the grand-daughter of Siu Chuang-ch'i.

K'ang Hsi, anxious for details of all the Western sciences, was also interested in medicine. In 1692 he had been cured of a malarial attack with a decoction of quinine prepared by two priests, Gerbillon and Pereyra, and in 1699 Frère Bernard Rhodes cured him of cardiac palpitations and boils on his upper lip. By his command Père Bouvet began a collection of anatomical charts, a task which was continued by Père Parennin (1665–1741) who composed in Manchu (probably between 1698 and 1722) a manuscript work on medicine, one copy of which, sent on 1 May 1723 to the *Académie Royale des Sciences*, is now in the library of the Paris Museum of Natural History. The book is in eight volumes, four being devoted to anatomy, three to pathology and the last to matters of physique and a few illnesses peculiar to women. The anatomical section was based on books by Pierre Dionis (Paris,

120

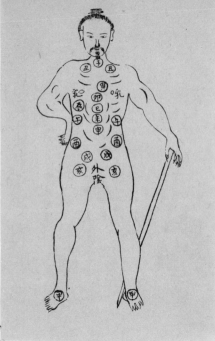

Illustrations from the first
work in Chinese devoted to
Western anatomy: the *Tai-si
jen-shen shuo-kai* ('Western
treatise on the structure of
the human body'), by Johannes
Schreck, otherwise Terenz or
Terentius (Chinese: Teng Yu-han,
c. 1576–1630?).

1690) for the text and Thomas Bertholin (Leyden, 1677) tor most
of the diagrams (118 out of 175). Parennin probably performed
several dissections, but there is no proof of this. His work carried
that of J. Schreck to a happy completion, adding to it the idea of
the circulation of the blood and lymphatic vessels.

K'ang Hsi was the more struck by European anatomical teaching
in that he had for several years acquainted himself with Western
medicine by having extracts from the reports of the *Académie
Royale des Sciences* 'dressed up in Tartar fashion' by Père Parennin.
He had decided on the advantage of 'dissecting those condemned
to death, who would thus compensate society for the wrongs they
had done'. But K'ang Hsi changed his mind. Not only did *Manchu
Anatomy* have no place in the scientific collections issued by the
Imperial press, but the right to read it was granted only to a
privileged few who were not allowed to borrow it or to take notes.
The book, he held, was exceptional; it could not be treated like
ordinary books nor left to the discretion of the ignorant. Thus
Manchu Anatomy, which in 1723 might have caused the stir

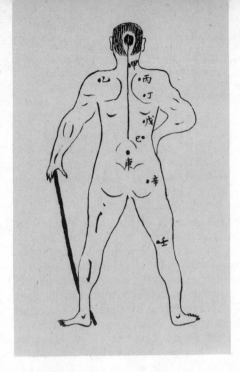

甲
乙 丙
丁
戊
己
東
辛

壬

produced in Japan in 1774 by the *Kaitai shinso*, had no influence on Chinese medicine.

Many Jesuits, among them Père Pierre-Martial Cibot (1727–80) and in particular Père Jean-Joseph Marie Amiot (1718–93), studied the book on the spot.

Further information has been left by several naval surgeons. Charles Gustave Ekeberg (1716–84), a Swedish doctor, naturalist and navigator, went to Canton in 1744 and from 1751 to 1754. He sent tea seedlings to Linnaeus and to the Uppsala botanical garden. He wrote articles on the metal tutenag, on the preparation of soya and oil, on the Chinese method of hatching ducks' eggs in ovens, and other topics.

Louis Relian (1726–73), a Genevan surgeon of the Dutch East India Company, studied in Paris and travelled twice to the Far East in 1752–4 and in 1770. He arrived at Canton in the *Overnez* and wrote a journal in French which was the subject of an article in the *Revue de l'Ecole d'Anthropologie* in 1904.

Andreas Sparmann (1747–1820), Professor of Natural History at

Page from Père Parennin's *Manchu Anatomy*. The Emperor K'ang Hsi was interested in Western medicine, and commissioned a collection of anatomical charts which Parennin completed in 1722. However, this work (which might have revolutionised Chinese anatomical thinking) was forbidden circulation and was not issued in the scientific collections from the Imperial press.

Uppsala, accompanied Captain James Cook on his voyage round the world. He visited China (1766) and the Cape (1772–5) and explored Africa, relating his travels in *Voyage to the Cape of Good Hope, to the South Polar Circle and round the world, including the country of the Hottentots and the Kaffirs* (1787).

East-West medical exchange A number of questions which were the subject of topical discussion among eighteenth century doctors in the West were already well known in Chinese medicine. Examples of these were the treatment of venereal disease, the diagnosis and prognosis of disease through the pulse, variolation, *materia medica*, acupuncture and cauterisation by moxas, and animal magnetism.

1 Jean Astruc (1684–1766) was the first European venereologist to add to his six hundred bibliographical references Chinese references drawn up by Père Pierre Foureau (1700–49), Père Dominique Parennin, Frère Rousset, and J. F. Vandermonde, a doctor at Macao from 1720 to 1723. He was so meticulous as to reproduce the Chinese medical characters referring to syphilis, the first venture of its kind in the West. He subsequently gave the text of the questionnaire he sent to Peking in 1737 and to which he received the first reply in 1739. This appeared in the fourth edition of his book on venereal diseases (1777). In 1737 Père Parennin sent a letter on venereal diseases in China to the St Petersburg Academy of Sciences which came into the possession of Antonio Nunès Ribeiro Sanchès (1699–1793), a physician to the Russian court. Astruc accepted the American origin of the pox and its transmission to the East and Far East by Europeans. For him the remarkable resemblance of the different therapeutic methods throughout Eurasia were an indication of the single source of the disease. Sanchez (Sanchès) on the other hand supported the theory that syphilis existed in Europe before Columbus.

2 Sphygmological diagnosis of disease was another bridge between the medicines of Europe and China, since at both ends of Eurasia diagnosis and prognosis were effected by taking the pulse. Wang Shu-ho's *Mo-ching* ('Pulse Classic') was not composed

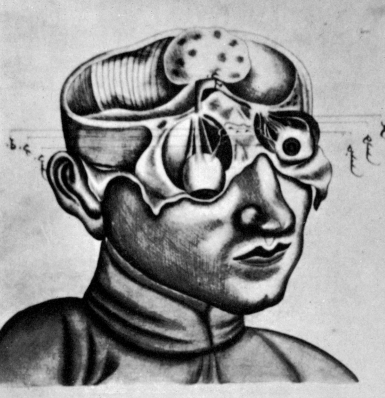

ولا حرف ك، دهه ككرد، وك بلا نتبه ::

نر :: تصييرين كتيبك دبك تسليمير سهم ::

نتبه :: تسييينيم كتيبك دبك تسليمير سهم ::

نتبه :: مبع دبك كتيبك دبك تسليمير سهم ::

كه :: تسيربك ديب، وك دبك سهم ::

كه :: تشيرين نك دييرين مبيرك سهم ::

نتبه :: تسيرسم دبك دبك تسليمير سهم ::

until the collapse of the Ancient Empire under the rule of the Western Chin dynasty (c. 265–316). We have seen how it had the good fortune to disclose the doctrine of the pulse to Tibetans, Indians, Koreans, Japanese, and Vietnamese. Thanks to the *Pax Mongolica* it had reached Istanbul; its last adventure was to bring it as far as Paris and London.

A French or French-speaking Jesuit missionary at Canton wrote the *Secrets de la Médecine des Chinois*, which was printed at Grenoble in 1671. Excluding works in Latin, this is the first Western work on the subject. The author, who has remained anonymous, wrote his preface at Canton on 21 October 1668. He must have been a French or Belgian missionary exiled by the Peking court to the banks of the Pearl River from 1665 to 1668. He is probably also the *eruditus europaeus*, the author of three letters written at Canton in 1669 and 1670 which are reproduced in the work of Andreas Cleyer. There is no mention of his sources, one of which was probably the *Nei-ching*.

The *Secrets*, translated into Italian (1676) and English (1707), attracted little attention. This was not however the fate of the *Specimen medicinae sinicae, sive opuscula medica ad montem sinensium* (Frankfurt, 1682), nor of the *Clavis medica ad chinarum doctrinam de pulsibus* (Nuremberg, 1686) and the *Secret du Pouls* (part of the *Description de la Chine*, 1735, by Père du Halde, 1674–1743).

The *Specimen* was compiled by Cleyer (1615–90) from heterogeneous documents belonging to Père Boym (1612–59), Eberhard Rumphius (1627–1702) and the mysterious exile of Canton. The original manuscript came into the hands of Christian Mentzel (1622–1701), physician to the Margrave of Brandenburg, and is today preserved in Berlin. Its sources were the *Nei-ching* (State Library) and the *Mo-kiue* ascribed to Wang Chu-ho. The *Clavis medica* is a very different work from the earlier *Specimen* dealing with the same subject. It is entirely the work of Boym, whose manuscript was given to Andreas Cleyer towards the end of 1681. Cleyer took it to Germany and had it published as an appendix to the proceedings of the *Academia Naturae Curiosorum*. The *Clavis*, which was again drawn from the *Nei-ching* and Wang Chu-ho, caused great interest both in medical spheres and among all those in Europe who belonged to the 'Republic of Letters'.

The *Secret du Pouls*, which was included in du Halde's monumental work, was by Père Placide Hervieu (1671–1746). It was an adaptation, with commentary and notes, of a *Mo chiue* ('Secret of the Pulse') of the Sung period. It had a second French edition (The Hague, 1736), English editions (1736, 1738–41, 1742), one German (1747–9) and one Russian edition (1774–7). Known in Germany through a version by Johann Conrad Barckhausen, called Barchusen (1666–1723), it was translated into English by William Wotton (1660–1726) and used by Sir John Floyer (1649–1734) in the first edition of *The Physician's Pulse Watch* (1707) also in a second volume (1710). For Floyer the pulse was the touchstone of harmony in the microcosm, and he set the sphygmology of Wang Chu-ho and Galen on the same level. This fondness for qualitative speculation prevented *The Physician's Pulse Watch* from effecting that progress in medical practice which might have been brought about by a quantitative and objective sphygmology. There was the same fundamental error in the revolutionary ideas which De Luques (1685–1738), De Bordeu (1722–76) and Fouquet (1727–1806) tried to bring to pulse symptomatology. The two Montpellier doctors were manifestly influenced by the Chinese technique. The observations of their Parisian rival Saillant (1747–1814) and Père Amiot left this fact in no doubt, as Professor Grmek has shown.

The theses which Abel Rémusat (1788–1832) and his friend Lepage defended in 1813 were the last flickers of Chinese symptomatology in French medicine. It may be observed however that Lepage's thesis was preceded by that of Bridault (*Medicinae sinensis conspectus*, *Monspelii*, 1759), who made his defence under the presidency of François Boissier de Sauvages (1706–67). It contained a short comparison of the Chinese doctrine of the pulse with Bordeu's theory.

With the review of several famous trials by the medical expert Antoine Louis, forensic medicine was very much in vogue. Père Cibot made a partial translation of the famous *Si-yuan-lu* and an index of it was inserted in the *Mémoires concernant les Chinois*.

3 The curious and edifying letters contained many details of the Chinese technique of variolation. A fine hand-painted album gave sixty-two portraits of children suffering from smallpox (*Bibliothèque Nationale*, *Cabinet des Estampes*, Oe 168).

Chinese surgery was of interest to the *Académie Royale de Chirurgerie*, and the subject was studied by two of its members: Dujardin (1738–75) and Pierre Süe (1739–1816). Dujardin based his work on Kaempfer; Süe drew his information from Père Raux (1754–1801) to whom he sent a questionnaire in 1786. Such cross-fertilisation belonged to an age in which D. Cassini and Joseph Nicolas de Lisle (1688–1768) questioned Père Gaubil (1689–1759) on the subject of Chinese astronomy, and in which Jean Rodolphe Perronet (1708–94), the famous engineer who built the *Pont de la Concorde*, made enquiries about Chinese methods of canal and garden construction.

4 *Materia medica* was mentioned in the general works of Du Halde (1730) and Moyriac de Maillac (1779). It was also the subject of a manuscript by Père d'Incarville now in the *Bibliothèque Nationale* (*Correspondance du Bréquigny*, Vol. 2). The Chinese *materia medica* was very badly documented by the West during this period; the word 'China' was associated with drugs which came not from Asia, but from America, like *Cortex-chinae*, a forgotten name for quinine. There was no lack of mistaken identifications. In common with its European counterpart of this period, the Chinese *materia medica* included the idea of the specificity of medicines, the doctrine of signatures, a fairly similar classification of therapeutic agents, and a certain number of basic medicines and therapeutic formulas.

Li Shih-chen was known through Du Halde's partial translation (1731) and through the *Dissertation sur l'origine, la dénomination et la curation des maladies vénériennes à la Chine* (Jean Astruc, third French edition 1775). Jacques François Vandermonde practised at Macao between 1720 and 1731, where he married in 1724. He returned to France in 1732 with his son Charles Augustin (1727–62), founder of the *Journal de médecine, chirurgie et pharmacie*.

Vandermonde brought back a translation of the mineralogical section of Li Shih-chen's *Pen-ts'ao chang-mu* (1593). It was accompanied by samples of the Chinese mineral *materia medica*, identified by Alexandre Brongniart (1770–1847) and studied by Edouard Constant Biot (1803–50) from 1835 to 1840. Vandermonde died in Paris in 1746. He had been one of Jean Astruc's sources of information, and many facts relating to medicine which we have already mentioned were to be found in his famous memoirs on the Chinese (1776–91) and in the correspondence of Henri Léonard Jean-Baptiste Bertin (1719–91) and Louis-Georges Oudard Feudrix de Bréquigny (1714–94). These were the subject of articles by E.C.Biot (1803–50) from 1835 to 1840.

Kaolin was discovered in western Europe by Darnet (at Saint-Yrieix) in 1771, thanks to the work of Pierre-Joseph Odolant-Desnos (1722–1801) and Jacques Etienne Guettard (1715–86).

At the beginning of the eighteenth century a number of herbal products used by the Chinese (ergot, chaulmoogra, *Ephedra*) were unknown in Europe, and were introduced only later in the century.

Canane (1764) and Odier (1774) restored castor oil to a place of honour, but they did not know that with alum and sugar the Chinese could remove its purgative property and make it edible.

Chinese rhubarb was the subject of much study on the part of Père Parennin (1727), Boerhaave (1750), and Linnaeus, who identified it as *Rheum palmatum*. Coste d'Arnoba imported some to the district round Paris (1777) and Desbarres to Brittany (1787), but it was not until about 1868 that H.Baillon, working on samples brought in by Dabry de Thiersant (1826–98), identified true pharmaceutical rhubarb (*Rheum officinale*), known to the Chinese by the name *Ta-huang*.

Geoffroy, who taught Père Chéron d'Incarville, carried out experiments in therapeutics with Japan wax.

128

The first Western mention of tea was by Giovanni Battista Ramusio (1485–1557) of Venice, and it was first featured in illustrations by W. Ten Rhyne (*c*.1683). Tea reached Holland in 1610, Paris in 1636, Moscow in 1659 and London in 1650, or possibly forty years earlier in 1606.[2] The first medical thesis devoted to the beverage was by Armand Jean de Mauvillain, a godson of Richelieu and was defended under the presidency of Philibert Moriset (*An the Chinesium menti confert?*). It was the subject of lively criticism between Guy Patin and his friend Spon of Lyons.

The plants and flowers of China in general were the subject of many articles by Gaubil, Parennin, Cibot, and especially Chéron d'Incarville who was the only missionary to be also a really competent botanist. His herbal of Chinese plants is in the phanerogamic laboratory of the Paris Museum of Natural History which, together with the library of the *Société Asiatique*, also has a replica of his manuscript album of Chinese plants. Other albums, produced at Peking by anonymous Chinese artists or by missionaries of this period, are in the library of the *Institut de France* and the *Bibliothèque Nationale*. All these unpublished works were the source of a herbal printed in colour (1781) which was compiled by Pierre Joseph Buchoz (1731–1807). João de Loureiro (1715–94) in his *Flora Cochinchinensis* (1790) described six hundred and eighty Chinese species observed for the most part in Macao and Vietnam. Another Chinese herbal was in the possession of the Abbé Tersan at the *Abbaye-aux-Bois*, and it was by studying this that J. P. Abel Rémusat became a sinologist before finishing his medical studies.

Magnificent albums, most of them in the Museum of Natural History, contained pictures of fish (the famous scroll of gold-fish), birds with flowers and insects, and also mammals. There are replicas in the *Cabinet des Estampes* of the *Bibliothèque Nationale*.

Musk and stag's horn were known in Europe as in China. Glue made from donkey-skin was the subject of a work by Parennin, author of the *Manchu Anatomy*.

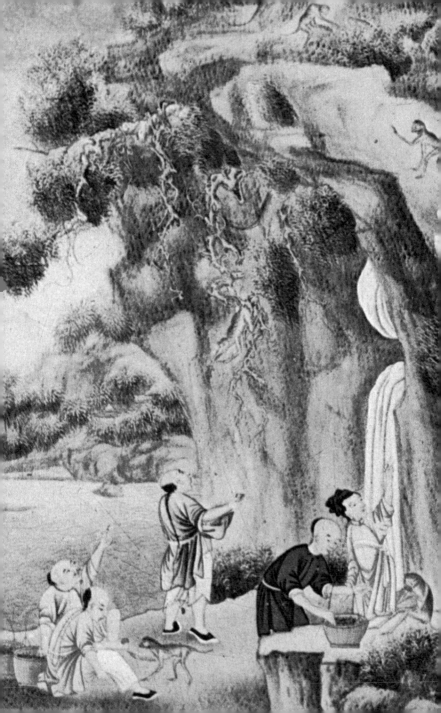

5 Acupuncture was first mentioned in the sixteenth century by Fernand Mendez Pinto, but it did not become generally known until the appearance of books by Ten Rhyne (1683) and Kaempfer (1712), surgeons of the Dutch East India Company, based on their observations in Japan. Félix Vicq-d'Azyr (1748–94) was the first French author after Dujardin to mention this form of therapy. We have already seen how actual cauteries of carded cotton came to Europe after their use in Egypt by Prosper Alpini (1553–1617), Johann Vesling (1610–49), and Dominique Larrey (1766–1842).

At the beginning of the seventeenth century there came news of the method of Japanese moxas ('the herb which burns') which Kaempfer Latinised as *moxibustio*. Ten Rhyne, Kaempfer, Hermann Buschoft, Andreas Cleyer, George Wedel, Karl Peter Thunberg praised this 'great incomparable' remedy. Fire therapy, dear to the Arabs and then expressly condemned at the beginning of the seventeenth century, thus came back into fashion at the end of the following century with Pouteau (1725–75), Percy (1790) and Larrey (1819). No further mention of the method appears in medical works after 1830.

6 Mesmer's doctrine of animal magnetism had hardly reached Peking when Père Amiot made a study of it in connection with the Taoist theories, accentuating certain similarities between mesmeric and *Tao-shih* (Taoist masters) practices. He developed the conception of a hydraulic and pneumatic physiology taken up by Dabry de Thiersant and Maspéro and finally, in a correspondence with C. Saillant (1747–1814), he gave a full commentary on Chinese sphygmology.

Amiot published an illustrated work on Taoist physiotherapy (*Chung-fu*) which probably helped to bring about the rebirth of European interest in physical culture. Similarities existing between the exercises he described and those of P. H. Ling (1776–1839), the founder of Swedish gymnastics, have been observed by Matignon and Needham. If we take into account the vogue of *Chinoiserie* in Sweden at the end of the eighteenth century, the hypothesis is a plausible one.

We may therefore conclude that, at the end of the *Ancien Régime* in France, Chinese medicine was fairly well known in Europe, especially in Parisian medical circles. It is no surprise to see that the first occupant of the Chair of Sinology at the *Collège de France* (1814) was a doctor, Jean-Pierre Abel Rémusat (1788–1832), whose 1813 thesis was on the Chinese practice of examining the tongue.

The nineteenth century

The eighteenth century had ended with the triumph of *Chinoiserie* in Europe. In China the light of Western science had reached the Forbidden City itself. Yet Europeans, for all their previous admiration of China earlier in the eighteenth century, now saw this, the greatest empire ever known and long reputed to be the most civilised, as nothing more than a despotic pagan state which the great powers were in duty bound to put down by military force. Convinced of their technical, military and scientific superiority, they could not imagine the existence of a standard of values other than their own and they regarded its manifestation in China as an example of bad taste. Conversely the Chinese viewed the West as inhabited by maritime barbarians more dangerous than the overland variety held back by the Great Wall, whom it was right to exclude from the Empire. It was in this difficult atmosphere, relaxed occasionally by the warmth of friendly relations between individuals, that European medicine took root in China.

British and American doctors After the opening of the treaty-ports, British and American Protestant missionaries, together with surgeons from the East India Company, took over from their Jesuit predecessors the task of initiating the Chinese to Western medicine. Spectacular successes in the field of therapeutics, the establishment of a scientific terminology, and the founding of schools and hospitals all helped towards the spread of Western ideas.

Individual European therapeutical successes can be listed as follows: Jennerian vaccination (1805), first amputation of the leg (Canton, 1836), first general anaesthesia by ether (Canton, 1847), first embryotomy (1858), first female lithotomy (Canton, 1874), first ovariotomy (Canton, 1875), first Listerian application (Shanghai, 1876). As was the case in the Middle East and India at this time, one of the main objectives in the Far East was the introduction of a scientific and medical terminology suitable for communications between China, Japan, and the West. Chinese translations of Western works were frequently adapted for Japanese and formed the basis of glossaries from Japanese into European languages, which were in turn retranslated into Chinese. Moreover, Japan was the country where many Chinese students went to learn the new medicine.

This linguistic work begun by the Jesuits and their Chinese associates was continued by the Protestant medical missionaries (Devan, 1847; Faber and Lobscheid, 1861; Hobson, 1887) and has not yet been brought to completion. The second objective was the publication of medical works, many of which came from the 'College for a Single Language' (*T'ung-wen chuan*). The final task was the foundation of schools for midwives, nurses, male nurses and doctors, and the building of hospitals. The missionary establishments were succeeded by private, governmental, and foreign secular establishments, but they were often ill-equipped and it was preferable for students to be sent abroad.

Among the earliest Western missionary and secular doctors we may note the names of Alex Pearson (1780–1874), Thomas Colledge, F.R.S. (1797–1879), a pupil of Sir Astley Cooper, 'Friend of the Chinese' and the founder of medical missions, Peter Parker (1804–88), American doctor and diplomat, W. Lockhardt (1814–96), the Rev. W. Burns (1815–68), Benjamin Hobson (1816–73), doctor and missionary of the London Missionary Society, translator of works on medicine and natural history. At Canton in 1851 he produced an anatomical atlas (*Ts'iuan-t'i sin-lun*), which was included in the collection *Hai-shan hien-chuan ts'ung-shu* by P'an Shih-ch'eng, printed from 1845 to 1849, and again in 1851 to 1885. This book reproduced part of the *Anatomical Tables* of William Cheselden (1688–1752) and was adapted in Japanese with the title *Zentai Shinron* by Gonzai Miyake (1852). Besides this summary of anatomy and physiology, illustrated by local artists (1851), he produced the following in Chinese: *A New Natural History* (1855), *Compendium of Western Medicine* (1857), *Obstetrics and Children's Diseases* (1858), *Comments on Internal Medicine* and *Anglo-Chinese Medical Vocabulary* (Shanghai Mission Press, 1858).

To James Henderson (*d.* 1865) were accredited the first autopsies, the first anatomical demonstrations (Shanghai, 1861) and the first lectures on post mortem examination technique to Chinese practitioners. J. G. Kerr (1828–1901), who succeeded Peter Parker, founded the Western Healing News (*Si-i sin-pao*) at Canton in 1881, the oldest Chinese medical journal written in Chinese, which ran to only nine issues. Other names to be mentioned are the Rev. Ernst Faber (1839–99), the Rev. Dyer Ball (*d.* 1866) and Cecil Davenport, F.R.C.S. (1863–1926). John Kenneth Mackenzie (1850–88) was the great surgeon of the English missions and performed a successful operation on Madame Li Hung-chang (1879).

Dudgeon, Professor of Medicine at the Imperial College, published an *Essay on Western Medicine* (1875), an *Illustrated Physiology* (1886), an *Anatomical Atlas* and a monumental *Anatomy* (twenty volumes, 1887).

Sir James Cantlie (1851–1926), Dean of the Hong Kong College of Medicine after Sir Patrick Manson, became the teacher and friend of Sun Yat-sen who was one of the first Chinese graduates of Hong Kong. Manson (1844–1922) carried out his fundamental research on the transmission of filariosis by mosquitos at Takao, Amoy and Hong Kong between 1866 and 1889. In 1894 he surmised that malaria was carried in a similar way, a theory which was proved by Sir Ronald Ross. His brother David, also a doctor, died in China in 1878. The reputations of S. W. Bushell, Robert

Morrison (the first translator of the Bible into Chinese), and W.A.P.Martin were well established by the end of the nineteenth century. By now many were aware of the possible transformation which might one day take place in the Empire, and in 1856 the Rev. W.A.P.Martin wrote:

We may certainly predict that if the T'ai-p'ing [rebel exponents of a popular uprising based on quasi-Christian ethics] continue to have the good fortune to be led by rulers as capable as those who have governed them until now, two or three years from the present time will be sufficient to make them masters of the Empire.

It was the British who set about the first general medical inquiry in China ordered by the Emperor T'ung Chih. It was led by Sir Robert Hart (1835–1914), Inspector-General of Customs (1863). He was a man of rare energy but despotic methods which caused his protégés to be nicknamed 'the royal family'. Each year he had Trade Reports published in which there was a section devoted to medical articles, and he in fact took over the running of the medical service. He lived in Peking, leaving from 1868 the duties of Inspector at Fuchow to Edgar. The most important treaty-port medical posts were held by Englishmen: Dudgeon in Peking (1865), William Gauld at Swatow (1863), F.Porter Smith at Hankow (1804), James Maxwell at Tachu (1864), MacGowan at Shanghai (1866), James Watson at Niou-chang (1865), John Frazer at Tientsin (1868), Brereton at Chefoo (1877), Reid at Hangchow (1870), Underwood at Kiukiang (1881). The 1,490 Chinese employed in the customs service of their own country were kept to fourth or fifth-grade duties of an anonymous kind.

Gutzlaff (1832), Hanbury (1862), Henderson (1864), Porter Smith (1871), MacGowan (1874), Thomson (1890) and Bretschneider (1894) produced some of the more noteworthy of the many publications in English on the subject of Chinese medicine.

Many military and Royal Navy surgeons came to China during the Opium War and the years which followed.

John Wilson, a naval surgeon and the founder of the Health

Report Annuals (1830–6), wrote in his *Medical Notes on China* (1846) about the beginnings of the colony of Hong Kong and the many psychological conflicts which set the Chinese and the 'red-haired barbarians' against each other.

A doctor in the Royal Navy who invited some Chinese doctors to be present at the autopsy of two English sailors received a note of thanks saying, 'We are overcome by your great kindness, but we must confess that everything we have just seen is in complete disagreement with the teaching of our books'.[3]

French doctors Despiau (*d.* 1824) arrived in Cochin China in 1789 and spent twenty years as physician to the court of Annam. In 1820 he went to Macao in search of anti-smallpox vaccine and attempted to introduce vaccination in Vietnam. In 1826 the *Héros* docked at Canton. On board was a surgeon working for the humble salary of one hundred francs a month, but who was later to become famous as the French Consul at Mosul where he made his reputation as an archaeologist. This was Paul Emile Botta (1802–70) who, after operating on a wounded sailor, returned to France in 1829 with entomological and botanical collections. Many more French boats came and moored at the quays of Canton in the nineteenth century, particularly frigates and store-ships voyaging on the great scientific circumnavigations. Their ship's doctors were sometimes eminent men, as for example Charles Gaudichaud-Beaupré (1789–1864), who during his voyage to Canton in 1837 learnt of his election to the botanical section of the *Académie des Sciences*.

Auguste Liautaud, a naval surgeon, called at Manila and Canton. In 1844 he sent a memorandum to the *Académie des Sciences* on Indian hemp and a copy of a Chinese anatomical chart. The Franco–Chinese War of 1885 brought many army and naval surgeons to the Far East. The chief medical officer of these troops was Didiot (*d.* 1903), who had under him a staff of about forty officers (doctors, surgeons, pharmacists and veterinary surgeons), among them being Duchêne (*d.* 1903), Guiliano, Guerrier, Armand

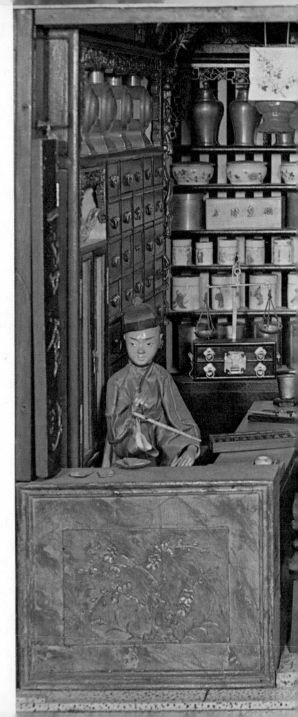

136

A model of a nineteenth-century pharmacy in Canton. The open front is typical. At the rear is an altar to the god of medicine, where incense was often burnt. The drug containers are of pewter and porcelain. The bearded proprietor serves tea to two customers, while in the foreground an assistant grinds drugs on a foot-operated mortar; other assistants weigh drugs.

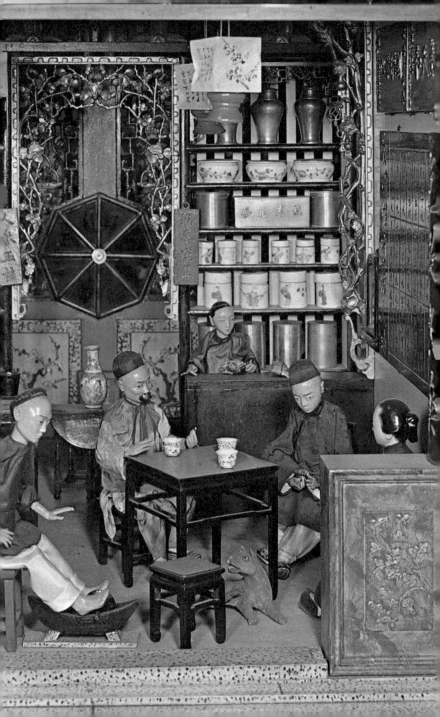

(author of letters on China to the *Gazette Médicale de France*), Champenois (*d.* 1890), Libermann (*d.* 1890), and the pharmacist Debeaux who in 1866 published a study of Chinese dyeing processes.

An infantry captain and later diplomat named Dabry de Thiersant (1842–98) served at Canton. He deserves mention for his work with Soubeiran (1827–92) on *La Médecine des Chinois* (1863) and *Matière médicale des Chinois*. The latter was the subject of a report by Gubler (1821–79) to the *Académie de Médecine* (1872) which resulted in 1874 in its publication at government expense. Dabry's careful research was recognised by Maspero, but his work has been used without acknowledgment by many writers on acupuncture.

Many naval surgeons spent some time at Shanghai, and some of them incorporated their Chinese observations into later theses: Lallemand, of the corvette *Constantine*; Le Tersec, of the corvette *Capricieuse*; Texier; Dumas; Le Coniat; all these wrote theses for Montpellier University in the period 1859–66.

François Sabatier (1822–67), on active service from 1859 to 1863 after running the naval hospital at Shanghai, wrote a thesis on the medical topography of Shanghai in 1864. Louis Marie Michel Toye (1824–1914) served for three years in China, meeting Père Vernez in 1854, who gave him several acupuncture charts and a manuscript on Chinese surgery ascribed to Jean Siu (*c.*1654). These documents are now kept in the library of St Anne's Hospital, Toulon, and were the subject of Toye's inaugural thesis (Montpellier, 1864).

The establishment of French diplomatic services led to the creation of consular medical posts. The first French diplomat (1845) to serve at Shanghai, de Lagrené, had with him a doctor by the name of Melchior Yvan (1805–73). After his return from China, Yvan taught at the Marseilles *École de Médecine* where he was Inspector-General of the press and the library. Alone and with the interpreter Callery he made a number of notes on Chinese medicine and pharmacy.

Georges Auguste Morache (1837–1906), a surgeon in the navy

and later a teacher of medicine at the University of Bordeaux, wrote about the foot deformities of Chinese women when in Peking and produced a report on Chinese medicine which was presented to the *Académie de Médecine*.

Jean-Jacques Matignon (1866–1928) first stayed in China as doctor to the colonial forces from 1894 to 1898. During that time he set up a hospital and the beginnings of a French school in Peking, and then studied the plague raging on the Mongolian and Siberian frontiers. He discovered unsuspected endemic centres and played a part in putting down the scourge which earned him the Russian Cross of St Anne. In 1895 he did distinguished work in the typhus, cholera and plague epidemics which claimed more than fifty thousand victims in Peking. A new outbreak of plague took him to Macao in 1897. After returning to France Matignon had no hesitation in setting out for Peking with the Allied forces for a second period from 1899 to 1901. While the legation was under siege he was taken for dead and the *British Medical Journal* published a premature obituary notice.

A brilliant journalist and observer, he studied Mongol medicine and the appalling social conditions of Peking at that time. His travel accounts give a description of the Ch'ing empire from the outsider's point of view, for he was not in fact a great expert on China.

Several French doctors worked for the Imperial Customs Service and in the teaching of medicine. Louis Pichon was one of 1,200 foreign agents of the Imperial Maritime Customs. He wrote for the first issues of the *Chinese Medical Journal* and practised at Shanghai from 1860 to 1905.

Under the Emperor Kuang Hsü a school of Western medicine (*I-hiue Chuan*) was founded at Tientsin in 1881 and reorganised by Li Hung-chang under the name of Pei-yang School of Medicine. The first principal was Li Lien-huei (1862–1900). One of his colleagues was Depasse (1859–1901), a naval doctor who had already served in Cambodia and Vietnam and had sailed in Admiral Courbet's squadron. He was temporarily released for service in Peking in 1894. With Li Lien-huei he attended Li Hung-chang and extracted a terrorist bullet which had lodged in his face. This earned him a vice-regal decree appointing him to succeed the English army doctor Houston in 1897 as Principal of the Pei-yang School. He later took the overland route back to France, travelling with Monnier from Peking to Ulan Bator in a palanquin. He died at an early age soon after his return.

Charles Louis-Maxime Durand-Fardel (1815–99), a well-known gerontologist and specialist in thermal treatment, was at Canton from 1875 to 1876. He brought back several articles on pathology and Chinese medicine and later became a member of the *Académie de Médecine* after writing in 1877 a survey on health conditions in China.

Yersin (1863–1943) explored the mountainous jungles of the three frontiers district (Vietnam, Laos and Cambodia) from 1890 to 1893. He was about to leave for Yünnan and had made contact with Dr Pichon of Shanghai when an epidemic of plague broke out, claiming sixty thousand victims in southern China. Owing to the departure of a colleague, Yersin was the only Pasteurian free to go to Hong Kong. He arrived in the epidemic area at the same time as Kitasato (1852–1931), exceptionally well-staffed and equipped. By repeated haemocultures Kitasato isolated a germ (quite different from the one found by Yersin) which he regarded as the agent of the plague until as late as 1899. In all probability it was a pneumococcus often associated with the plague bacillus and concealing it by its proliferation.

From June to August of 1894 Yersin made his name by looking for the plague bacillus in the buboes rather than the blood and by reproducing the disease experimentally, which his Japanese rival had not succeeded in doing. He easily obtained pure cultures which were verified in Paris. On 30 July he reported his discovery to the *Académie des Sciences* and in the *Archives de Médecine Navale*.

Deblenne, a doctor of the mission from Lyons, passed through Canton (1895–8) on his way up to Kansu where he made ethnological notes on south-west China.

Cyprinus carpio (the *li-yu* or Chinese goldfish (*chin-yu*)). This famous scroll was sent to Paris in 1772 by a member of the Peking mission.

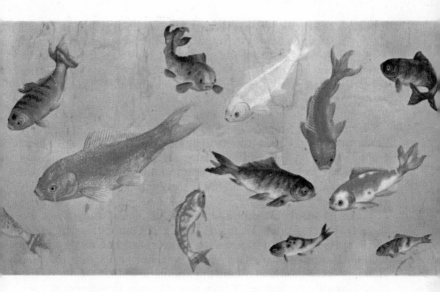

Maurel (1847–1918), a doctor in the navy who later taught at the Toulouse Faculty of Medicine, served in Cambodia and called at Canton.

Medical missionaries were few, all of them Jesuits: Père Rathouis (1834–90), a botanist and zoologist, sent specimens to the *Musée Heude*, while Père Chauvin (1823–1903), previously a naval surgeon, was Superior of the Chiang-nan Mission.

Leading French medical experts spoke highly of Chinese medicine. Gubler, Baillon and Soubeyran were interested in the *materia medica*. De Mély produced his *Lapidaires chinois* (1896) in collaboration with Courel. The Chinese member of the *Simarubaceae* family, *Ailantus glandulosa*, came into use for the treatment of dysentery. Mattei (1862) and Armand (1874) did a considerable amount of work on opium. Daremberg wrote in 1849:

142

Many a time, however, I have had the opportunity to make observations which show that, without claiming any remarkable cures, sensible unprejudiced men could derive immense profit from books on Chinese medicine if they were translated or abridged under the direction of a competent person. I have seen, for example, that the Chinese have long made use of pomegranate rind to destroy tapeworms, ergot to hasten difficult labour, substances containing iodine to cure goitre, warm salt water drunk in large amounts for cholera (a method approved last year by Russian doctors), etc.

For some years early in the nineteenth century, acupuncture enjoyed as great a French vogue as auscultation. The *Académie des Sciences* appointed a commission to study it, and clinicians like Cloquet and Trousseau were among those interested. After some decades, however, the method was forgotten, whereas Chinese medicine in general continued to be the subject of many works, such as those by Rémusat (1813), Lepage (1813), Bricheteau (1819), Julien (1849), Lecoq (1857), Briau (1857), Pauthier (1860), Larivière (1863), Gauthier (1863), Debeaux (1865), Bordier (1872), Daumas (1877), Verrier (1887) and Martin (1885).

The 'artificial paradise' of opium was known in Europe as early as the first quarter of the nineteenth century. But the most notable drug addicts, like De Quincey in England and Baudelaire in France, were eaters rather than smokers of opium. Opium smoking, originating probably in Iran and brought into the Far East by the Dutch in the eighteenth century, was practically unknown in Europe. The main contribution to a reappraisal of the therapeutic use of opium was made by doctors in the army and navy (Liautaud, Mattei, Libermann, Laborde, Armand, Martin) who also carried out the first medical survey of opiate poisoning by pipe-smoking.

Russian doctors Tatarinov (*d.*1886) was responsible for a number of published works reviewed in the *Medizinische Zeitung Russlands* (1853 and 1858). He produced the *Catalogus medicamentorum Chinensium, quae Pekini comparanda et determinanda curavit A. Tatarinov* (Petropolis, 1857). He also studied the circulation of the blood, anaesthesia, anatomy and physiology, and more especially the study of the *Pen-ts'ao*. Emile Bretschneider (1833–1901), a doctor at the Russian Legation in Peking, published important geographical and botanical works, one of them the *Botanicon Sinicon*.

The twentieth century

At the end of the First World War the established order (hitherto largely of a nineteenth century character) no longer could seem so solid and inevitable. The Second World War was even more disruptive for a Europe which had ceased to impose its own aims upon the world.

The taste in certain circles for the exotic, the mysterious and the superhuman; the loss of self-sufficiency vis à vis non-European civilisations; the fact that after the collapse of colonialism millions of Asiatics are gaining in demographic importance without recourse to an expensive and complicated scientific medicine – all these factors explain why Eastern medical systems today enjoy favour among Western patients and doctors. Another significant factor in the development of this new attitude, thanks to the efforts of orientalists in the last century, is the birth of a 'new humanism' whereby all civilisations are worthy of study. In this perspective, all medical systems no matter what their practical value have an equal interest in the eyes of the medical historian. The 'great rondure' of the world will not become reality until such an attitude informs every aspect of the art of healing, regardless of place and time. Then only will an atmosphere of mutual co-operation be possible, in which doctors from every part of the world will be at their ease. That is why Chinese medicine, so long scorned, occupies its rightful place in Sarton's *Introduction to the History of Science* (1, 1927; 2, 1931; 3, 1948), the reference book for all English-speaking science historians.

A final reason is the change in general medical opinion. Until about the first quarter of the twentieth century Western medicine was essentially an anatomo-clinical medicine in which symptoms referred always to macroscopic or microscopic lesions, revealed by autopsy or on microscopic sections. Virchow refused to be drawn into any discussion with those who acknowledged the existence of 'general illness'. Now that it has been proved that authentic diseases can be characterised not by lesions but by functional disturbances; now that medical psychology and psycho-somatic medicine have revealed to us the importance of psychological, moral and mental factors in the origin of disease and the behaviour of patients, new interest is taken in the old, obsolete medical systems with their non-anatomical foundations. It has also been noticed that the *materia medica* of distant lands (especially with regard to herbs) deserve systematic exploration.

French doctors Regnault (1873–1962) arrived in Vietnam in 1898 and began to learn to speak Mandarin and read Chinese characters. He studied the connection between the philosophy of the Chinese and their medical system, publishing the result of his research in 1902. With Irving Hancock he was one of the first Europeans to draw attention of the manual methods of resuscitation in use in Japan (*Kuatsu*).

Jeanselme (1888–1935), a graduate of the Paris Faculty of Medicine, was commissioned to study leprosy in the Far East. He visited Siam, Malaya, Vietnam, Cambodia, Laos, Burma and Yünnan. During the course of this mission he collected a considerable number of documents on exotic diseases (leprosy, beriberi, yaws, syphilis, smallpox, and mental disorders), toxicoses (opium addiction and alcoholism), anthropology, forensic medicine and the history of medicine.

Mesny (1869–1911) served first of all as a naval doctor in Senegal (1894–9). He transferred to the Colonial Forces and was later appointed successor to Depasse, as Principal of the Municipal School of Medicine at Pei-yang, to which the Viceroy Yüan Shih-K'ai looked for his first military doctors and pharmacists. Mesny was active in the struggle against the plague epidemics of 1903–4 and 1905, the epidemic of exanthematic typhus in 1904 and the cholera epidemic of 1907. In 1908 pulmonary plague broke out in the north of Manchuria, Harbin being a main centre of infection. Mesny rushed there, but fell a victim himself despite the ministrations of his Russian colleague Haffkin (1860–1930). France was greatly affected by the news of his death and a bust of Mesny was erected at Brest, his birth-place.

Legendre joined the naval medical section in 1889 later transferring to the Colonial Force. He found his true vocation as an explorer on eight expeditions to China and Indochina financed by the *Museum National d'Histoire Naturelle*, the *École d'Anthropologie* and the French Ministries of Education and Foreign Affairs in the first quarter of this century. In 1909 he made a study of the Lolo and Sifan tribes in China's western hill country which he reported to the *Société de Géographie*.

Legendre specialised in the Chinese minorities (in particular the Lolos). Jouvelet, who taught for a long time at the *École de Médecine*, and Jouveau-Dubreuil practised at Chengtu. There Jouvelet met Henry, with whom he constructed the first French blood transfusion apparatus to have extensive use. It was there also that Paris succeeded Jouvelet in 1923 and took over the direction of the Pei-men Vaccine Institute (*Pei-men wei-cheng-chia hang*). This mission included two naval doctors, Arnaud and Gervais. Both taught at the Military Medical School (*Chiun-i hiue-t'ang*) and were in attendance at the hospital of the Roman Catholic mission (*P'ing-an-chiao i-yüan*).

Béchamp, the son of the famous Montpellier chemist and opponent of Pasteur, was a doctor with the *Messageries Maritimes* and had learnt Chinese. He practised at Chengtu and then at Hangchow from 1928 to 1934. He died in Shanghai in 1945 at Japanese hands.

In 1912, with the help of prominent people like Ma Sian-tih and Lo Pah-hung, Ricou founded the medical department of the *Université Aurore* at Lo-ka-we, centring it on St Mary's Hospital (*Chuang-tzu i-yuan*, built in 1907). The first diplomas were awarded in 1917, and up to 1949 the French Faculty of Medicine at Shanghai was training between twenty-five and thirty doctors a year. Its influence spread over the whole of the Far East through its *Bulletin* and its Heude Museum (1942). Its teachers have included Florence (1917–23), Champonnière (1923–5), Porak (1923–5), Malval (1934–46), Martin (1935–45), and Flamet (1938–50). The *Aurore* Faculty of Medicine had 290 students on its roll in 1948.

Bussière (1872–1958) made a study of the thermal springs at Si-shan while in Peking. As Dean of the Faculty of Medicine of the *Université Aurore* from 1934 he regularly presided over examining boards at Shanghai. During the Second World War he retired to Peking but was obliged by circumstances to return to France.

Victor Segalen (1878–1919) made a voyage to Polynesia before serving in China. A qualified Chinese scholar, he taught at the Tientsin School of Medicine as successor to Mesny. He was also Yüan Shih-k'ai's personal physician from 1912 to 1913. After an archaeological expedition to western China with Jean Lartigue and Gilbert des Voisins he returned to the French front in 1915. He was an excellent musician, friend of Gide, Claudel, and Saint-John Perse, and wrote poems and an opera (*Orphée-Roi*) for which Debussy intended to write the music. As well as being essentially a poet, he was also philosopher, art critic, novelist, a most conscientious doctor and a successful archaeologist.

Segalen wrote a great deal, but some of his manuscripts were not published until after his death. A recent thesis by Henry Bouiller (1962) presents his bibliography and an excellent survey of his work. For Segalen man's noblest task was in trying to surpass himself, inspired by what theologians call a threefold libido: *libido sentiendi, libido sciendi* and *libido dominandi*.

His intellectual adventure was a 'quest for the unicorn', a pursuit of the 'fanciful' in which one delights, truer than reality with its rude shock, but passing over it and extending it and perhaps even going beyond it, the 'after-world'. The pursuit of the 'fanciful' is complemented by the pursuit of the 'changing', in which he shows himself to be more sensitive to the contrast of different objects than to the objects themselves. The 'changing' has its own aesthetics: exoticism (see his *Notes sur l'exotisme*, Mercure de France, 1955). 'Exoticism', he wrote, 'a word so often debased, is everything "other". To enjoy it is to learn the taste of the "changing".' Segalen was passionately concerned to restore to foreign countries and races their original importance. His own work reflects the 'exoticism' of long journeys to distant lands, as well as 'exoticism of time' demanding knowledge of the birth of civilisations. Thus in him the poet transcends the archaeologist. His exoticism was in the main Polynesian and Chinese. He gave Taoism a new form of linguistic and poetic expression.

Among the French who visited China there is one young man whose story is particularly interesting. One day a down-and-out Chinese was picked up on the quayside at Saint-Nazaire by Théophile Gautier who towards 1863 made him tutor to his daughter. She eventually introduced him to Georges Soulié de Morant, who, having in this way learnt some rudiments of Chinese as a young man, left for China. He served as consul and spent his leisure in the study of art and acupuncture. When he returned to France he advanced the cause of acupuncture in French medical circles with Flandrin and Ferreyroles. Soulié de Morant based his work essentially on the *Chen-chiou ta ch'eng* by Yang Chi-chou (*c.* 1657).[4]

Among French publications – of very uneven standard – dealing with Chinese medicine we may mention those by Vincent (1915), Regnault (1902), Perrot and Hurrier (1907), Leroy (1910), Matignon (1913), Doré (1920), Demiéville (1929), Maspéro (1937), Fautereau-Vassel (1939), Roi (1955), and Cassien Bernard (1957).

English and American doctors Mention should be made of the work of Porter Smith, revised by Stuart (1911), of Laufer (1919), Cowdry (1921), Dawson (1925), Read (1931–41), Morse (1934), De Sowerby (1934), Hume (1940), Veith (1949), Needham (1954), Hoeppli (1959) and Mann (1962). A special place must be given to a Canadian surgeon, Norman Bethune (1890–1939). He was in the ambulance service in France during the First World War and went to Spain in 1936 during the civil war. When China was invaded by Japan in 1937 he was one of the first to organise help in America for Chinese resistance. He went to China as a volunteer, was engaged on an advanced surgical shock unit, and reached Yenan in April 1938. The following June he successfully crossed occupied China and joined the resistance base of Shansi-Chahar-Hopei where he set up a model hospital (now the International Peace Hospital).

In 1939 he was transferred to a Hopei field-hospital where, in the midst of battle and under enemy fire, he operated in exceptional circumstances, exhausted and without even a pair of gloves. In this way he contracted septicaemia from contact with an infected wound. Completely incapacitated by the infection, he was evacuated by his own stretcher-bearers while under fire from the approaching enemy. He was particularly anxious to be taken back to his hospital unit where, in the great Chinese medical tradition, he died among his disciples. His story has been celebrated by a commemorative stamp, while a medical foundation, the Norman Bethune Medical School, has been established in his memory.

German doctors The German medical school at Shanghai was founded shortly before the First World War but did not survive the Second. Professors Fisher and Wagenseil taught there for a number of years. Mention should be made of the work of Gruenhagen (1908), Hübotter (1929 and 1957), Eckstein (1925), Heusinger (1931), Hartner (1942), Bachmann (1952), Stiefvater (1957), Schramm (1958), Wallnöfer and Von Rottauscher (1959) and Von Roques (1962).

Russian doctors Russian writers on Chinese medicine include: Bretschneider (1882), Matveyev (1903), Violin (1903), Kirillov (1914), Korsakov (1928), Marakuev and Rudanov (1935), Viazmensky (1955), Rossiisky (1951), Straschun (1955), Kochergin (1959), Ibraguimov and Ibraguimova (1960), and V.G. Vogralik (1961).

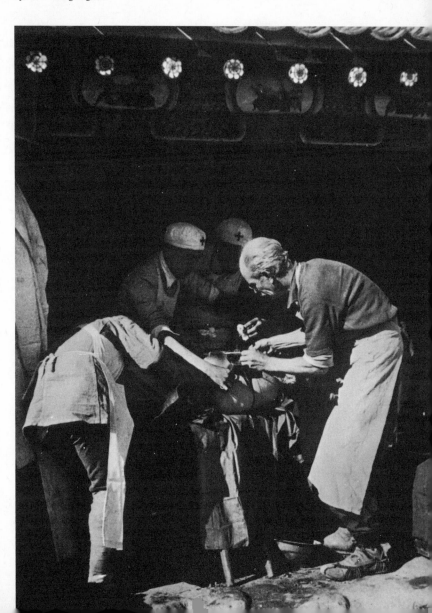

Dr Norman Bethune (1890–1939)
operating under battle conditions
during the Japanese war in China.
A medical foundation bearing
his name has been established
by the Peking régime.

A group of Soviet doctors completed a course of traditional medicine in Chinese hospitals (1956–7) and then practised *chen-chiou* therapy (treatment with needles and moxas) in institutions in the USSR including the Laboratory of Reflexotherapy. Moscow; the Laboratory of *Chen-chiou* Therapy of the Institute of Neurophysiology, Leningrad; the Department of Therapeutics at the Gorki Hospital; the Department of Diseases of the Nervous System at the Kazan Institute of Advanced Medicine; the Department of Therapeutics at the Armavir Hospital. All these schools made use of the methods of the Institute of Experimental Acupuncture directed by Madame Chu Lien (Peking).[5]

4 Western Medicine in modern China

The fall of the Ch'ing dynasty, long prepared in the south and by the outer provinces, was followed by the National Republic (1912–49) which was in its turn succeeded in 1949 by the People's Republic.

Works of Western influence

Several publications show that Western anatomy has continued to interest the Chinese. Yu Cheng-sie (1775–1840), in his *Kuei-szu lei-Kao* (1815), alluded to the structure of the human body (*Jen-shen t'u-shuo*) by Schreck, adapted by Pi Chung-ch'en (*d.* 1644) (see page 120).

Wang Shih-hiung (*c.* 1808–50) wrote *On Cholera*, *On Warmth and Heat*, *On Plagues and Malaria*, and *On Medical Cases*. He did not regard European medicine as the only one of value but recommended a mixture of the two schools. Yu Li-ch'u at about the same period tried to refute the *Jen-shen t'u-shuo* of Père Rho by referring to the comparative structure of the heart and the intestine in Europeans and Chinese. He held that the situation of the heart and liver was reversed in the two races, that their religion must therefore be different and that only Chinese who were organically inverted or incomplete could be converted to Christianity. He added ironically that if the Western missionaries were less ignorant they would not be wasting their time converting the abnormal and would go home.

Wang Ts'ing-jen, also called Wang Hiun-ch'en (1768–1831) wrote an *I-lin chai-tso* ('Corrector of Medical Errors') which caused as much stir in the medical world of 1797 as Liao P'ing's *Studies on the False Classics* did in literary circles. Wang Ts'ing-jen was born in the district of Yu-t'ien (Chihli) and devoted forty years of his life to the study of splanchnology and to refuting the errors of the *Nan-ching* ('Classic on Difficult Problems'). He was bent on correcting all the commentaries of the early writers and concentrated his findings in the small volume mentioned.

In the second year of the reign of Chia Ch'ing (1796–1820),

Wang, then aged thirty, went to the Luanchou district shortly after a cholera epidemic and found a number of children's corpses which had been given only superficial burial. The starving dogs prowling near the public cemeteries were digging up the corpses and provided Wang with the dissecting models with which to make his spectacular discovery of the errors of the early anatomists. He became enthusiastic over this new line of study and is thought to have dissected more than thirty corpses in ten days.

It is possible that he followed up his human dissections by dissecting animals.

He recorded his observations in twenty-four remarkable diagrams, drawn by himself and reproduced in his book. They present ideas which had until then escaped the writers of the classics:

1 the epiglottis, a continuation backwards of the base of the tongue through the trachea and its bifurcation ('left and right-hand gates of the breath');
2 the epiploon, where he located the 'central burner';
3 the ureter, the vas deferens;
4 the arch of the aorta, the thoracic aorta and the inferior vena cava;
5 the pancreas.

Wang was interested in the brain (categorised by the classics with the bone marrow) and the excretory passages for the urine. Unfortunately, just as Vesalius was unable to abandon certain tenets of Galenic philosophy and postulated imaginary organs, so Wang was unable to give the aorta, the vena cava and the ureter their true significance. It was psychologically impossible for him to achieve his end and correct all the errors in the *Nei-ching*. For him the kidney and its cords (the ureters) had an essentially genital function. The idea of urine secreted by the kidney and conveyed by the ureter to the bladder eluded him as completely as it did his pupil P'eng Tsung-hai.

P'eng Tsung-hai, a disciple of Wang Ts'ing-jen and a native of the Szechwan province, lived during the reign of Kuang Hsü (1875–1907) and wrote a comparative study of the Chinese and Western

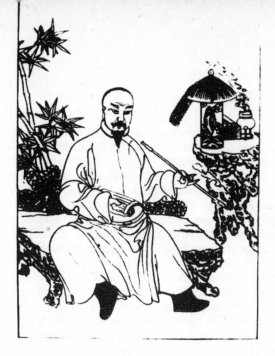

Wang Ts'ing-jen (1768–1831), an anatomist, therapeutist, and reformer of traditional medicine. His *Corrector of Medical Errors* of 1797 put right many of the mistaken assumptions of the early *Nan-ching* (the 'Classic on Difficult Problems').

medical systems (*Chung-si i-hiue huei-t'ung*, *c*. 1876). He had access to Western anatomical atlases and was thus able to compare them side by side with the data of the *Nei-ching*. Nevertheless he remained loyal to the tradition of Chinese scholars and wrote a commentary on the early theories. He again held that the 'cords' of the kidney corresponded to the gate of life (*Ming-men*) and that the fat under the cords represented the 'lower burner', the fat in the region of the omentum corresponded to the 'central burner', and the upper part of the diaphragm to the 'upper burner'. (It is known that some contemporary authors took the analogy further and compared the three burners to the lymphatic system). P'eng described the part of the bladder 'relating to the fat as the place where the water (i.e. the urine) enters'.

Lastly he was apparently convinced that the brain controls the action of the heart, which is in complete contradiction to the theories of Chin Cheng-si and Li Shih-chen, since the one held that the brain was the seat of the memory and the other that it was the 'Palace of God'.

Although he denied it, Wang Ts'ing-jen was a therapeutist as well as an anatomist and reformer of traditional medicine. He stated that 'diseases are countless and it is hardly possible to give a complete collection of them'. Above all he tried to give a correct picture of them. Thirty-three prescriptions (*fang*) can be taken from his work, two of them borrowed from early writers and dealing with gynaecology and pediatrics.

Chang Chung-ching (*c.* AD 200) was one of his sources. There is also evidence of the influence of Wang Ch'en-t'ang (1549–1613), the author of the most famous general medical work of the sixteenth century, the *Cheng-chih chun-shen*, of Prince Chou Ting (Chu Su), patron of the *P'u-tsi-fang* ('Prescriptions to Save the World') by T'eng Shuo, Liou Ch'un and others, and of Li Shih-chen. Wang Ts'ing-jen applied himself to the study of tonics to strengthen the breath (*pu-ch'i*) and, as we have observed, to disperse extravasate blood (*siao-yu*).

Another of his interests was the study of smallpox (*t'ien-hua*). Since the Han period certain authors held the theory of poison of the embryo (*t'ai-tu*). The *t'ai-tu* lay in the organs and viscera (*tsang-fu*) and made its appearance only during illness in the form of smallpox pustules. Others asserted that it was to be found in the bone marrow (*ku-suei*). He decisively refuted all these erroneous beliefs and emphasised the infectious, eruptive, contagious and epidemic nature of the disease. He described *wen-tu* (epidemic poisoning) in careful detail.

The *I-lin-chai-tso*, written *c.*1796–8, was not printed until 1850. Dudgeon, on the staff of the College for a Single Language (*T'ung-wen chuan*), is thought to have translated it into English in about 1893–4, referring to Wang as the modern Chinese anatomist.

Chinese doctors of Western influence

From 1806 Alex Pearson (1780–1874) had a Chinese assistant, Yau Ho-shun (You Ho-chuan, *d.*1850) who, with his son Yau Yam-teng, promoted Jennerian vaccination. He wrote a short work in Chinese on the subject in 1818.

Peter Parker trained Chuan A-to (1818–74), the first Western-type Chinese surgeon. He could be compared to Pandit Mad-husudan Gupta, the first Indian surgeon to carry out a surgical operation according to Western techniques (on 10 January 1836).

Wung Shuk-hing (Huang Ch'o-hing), otherwise called Wung Fun (Huang Ch'uan) (1828–78), the first Chinese to qualify abroad, a Doctor of Medicine of Edinburgh University, taught at the Canton School of Medicine where he carried out the first operations based on anatomical knowledge (first embryotomy in 1860). He travelled to the USA and eventually became medical adviser to Li Hung-chang (1823–1901). His example was followed by Sir Chai Ho-chai (1859–1914) and Madame Hu Chi-meng (1865–1929) (Hu Chin-ying), the first woman teacher at Fuchow.

So To-meng (1847–1919) went to America and became an ophthalmologist and anaesthetist. Lim Boon Keng (b. 1869), D.M. Edinburgh, wrote the first Chinese work on microbiology. He became president of the University of Amoy. Li Shu-fan (b. 1886), also an Edinburgh alumnus, was the director of the Kwangtung Health Service.

Women began to enter medicine in the last years of the century. Yamei Chin (b. 1864) became in 1885 the first Chinese woman to graduate abroad. She specialised in microphotography in New York. Mention must also be made of Mary Stone (b. 1873), Ida Kahn (1873–1931) and Mary Fulton (d. 1929), Principal of the Hackett Medical College for Women at Canton.

The next generation brought personalities like Wang Shung-yik (1888–1930), the first Professor of Pathology at Hong Kong, Tsegang F. Huang (1899–1940), an American-trained bacterio-logist and doctor, and Sung Tsai-pao (1907–40), a teacher at the Shanghai *Université Aurore*.

Towards the end of the nineteenth century there were about a hundred American and European doctors resident in China. Many were members of the Association of Medical Missionaries, formed in 1887, and readers of its *China Medical Missionary Journal* published at Shanghai. Others, as we have seen, were surgeons in

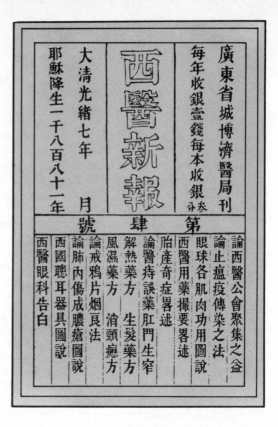

the Customs service. They took part in the medical service organised in every port open to foreigners. Every six months their work was reported in the form of bulletins published by the Inspector-General of Customs. Finally there were the private doctors of important personages, such as Drs Irwin and Mark in the service of the Viceroy Li Hung-chang. From 1883 onwards the Peking School of Medicine was turning out the first Western-trained Chinese doctors after a four-year course. One of them, Chin Ta-shin, was decorated by the emperor for services during the war between China and Japan.

It will be remembered that Western medicine was reintroduced in Peking by Lockhart who carried on the work begun by the Jesuit doctors in the eighteenth century. His successor, Dudgeon,

The first Chinese journal
devoted to Western medicine,
Western Healing News (1881).

157

worked in the hospital he had opened in 1861 and which formed
the nucleus of the Peking Union Medical College. This was shortly
before the birth in 1866 of Sun Yat-sen, also called Sun Wen or
Sun Chung-shan in the village of Tsuei Heng, near Macao in
Kwangtung province. After education at an Anglican school in
Honolulu, Sun became a Christian, returning to his native village
where he defied the old idols and caused such a scandal that he had
to flee to Canton. There he took a post in an Anglo-American
hospital for about a year.

He earned the good opinion of his employers, and when he
wanted to study medicine they allowed him to enter the Hong Kong
School of Medicine where he became the pupil and friend of Sir
James Cantlie (1851–1926), who wrote a biographical account
of him.

Meanwhile he had become reconciled with his family and had
even consented to marry in accordance with Chinese customs.
After five years' study (1892) he received his Diploma in Medicine
and opened a surgery at Macao. It was at this time that he took the
name Sun Yat-sen. Thereafter his career is part of the history of
modern China and of little medical interest. After exile in Europe
and America, he returned to Japan, where he organised the anti-
dynastic society known as the *T'ung-meng huei*, and then moved
to Hanoi to instigate numerous insurrections in south China.
Finally, in October 1911, one such uprising was successful, though
it was only later that Sun achieved real political power with his
Kuomintang party after the failure of Yüan Shi-k'ai's imperial
restoration. Sun Yat-sen died of cancer in 1925 and is buried in
Nanking.

Another well-known doctor was Wu Lien-to (1879–1959), a
native of Penang. He studied medicine in London where he made
a life-long friendship with E. E. Hume (*d.* 1957). He returned first
to Malaya and then soon afterwards went to China where he
entered the Imperial health service in 1908. He did distinguished
work in the Harbin plague epidemic of 1910 by the side of the
famous Russian epidemiologist Haffkin (1860–1930) and the

Frenchman Mesny. He was subsequently in charge of the quarantine service and represented his country at international conferences, was physician to state leaders, and contributed to the foundation of the *Academia Sinica*. His autobiography, and his *History of Chinese Medicine* which he wrote with K. C. Wong, show him to have been an ardent enthusiast for Western medicine.

Yu Shu-fen, head of the medical mission sent to Chihli, met his death in 1921 fighting the plague epidemic brought in from Manchuria.

Medical education

The teaching of medicine meanwhile was progressing. Chang Pai-hi drew up in 1902 the rules for schools of medicine designed for a course of three years. In 1903 the *Chin-shih-ta-hiue-t'ang* (University of Peking) opened a school of medicine, also with three-year courses. It became a Faculty of Medicine (*I-hiue chuan*) in 1905 with the help of Sun Chia-nai, Chang Chih-tung, Chang Pai-hi and Yung Ch'ing. The Chinese Red Cross began in 1904

As already noted, Yüan Shih-k'ai organised in 1901 the *Pei-yang* School of Medicine at Tientsin which provided the Chinese army with its first medical officers.

Ch'iu Yung-ts'iou founded the Canton School of Military Medicine in 1909, and in 1911 the Cho-Chiang Faculty of Medicine was opened with T'ang Ul-ho as its first principal.

Official regulations for the dissection of corpses were promulgated in 1913. Several important foundations after that date were: 1914, China Medical Board, through the Rockefeller Foundation; 1915, National Medical Association; 1923, National Yünnan University; 1927, School of Military Medicine (*Lu-Chiun i-hiue-hiao*) founded by Siu Hua-ching and later reorganised by Sun Liou-hi; 1923, *Academia Sinica* at Nanking and the National Academy of Peking, Fan Memorial Institute of Biology; 1937, Chinese Medical History Society; 1939, Yingshih University (Cho-chiang); 1930, first official pharmacopoeia.

Between 1921 and 1929 forty-five medical journals appeared, some of them lasting for several years. Many hospitals were built, partly by public subscription. Gradually a number of teaching centres were founded for nurses, male nurses, and midwives. As for the training of doctors, in 1916 there were twenty-six schools of medicine (thirteen of them missionary) with 1,940 students. In 1935 these numbers had risen to thirty-three Faculties of Medicine, 20,799 beds distributed over five hundred hospitals, 3,528 students and some fourteen to twenty thousand practitioners of Western influence (*si-i*) of which only seven thousand were thought to be registered.[1]

These numbers increased considerably until about 1940, when the Japanese invasion, the transfer of the northern universities southwards and the civil war made systems costly and difficult to work, while supplies of medicines, instruments and various kinds of equipment were problematical.

Many accounts give us an idea of the medical distress of this period, during which Bethune of Canada and Kotnis of India did distinguished work. Both died in their devotion to the service of the Chinese people.

By Liberation in 1949, the population of some six hundred million Chinese had been reduced by millions as a result of undernourishment, tuberculosis, cholera, schistosomiasis, typhoid, dysentery and a vast number of parasitic affections.

There were eighty-seven hospitals, the larger ones having a total capacity of some 6,400 beds. In Peking there were only 11,000 beds for three million inhabitants, and at Shanghai 17,000 beds for a population of seven million. Nearly a thousand health centres were built or restored to running order.

The number of Western-trained doctors fluctuated between twenty and thirty-five thousand, most of them qualified or having done special studies in America or in Europe. This gave a ratio of one modern doctor to 25,000 people, whereas in the developed countries one doctor is hardly sufficient for five to seven hundred people. Twenty thousand doctors (for a population bigger than that of the USA, the USSR and Europe combined) is only twice the total in Belgium.[2]

The peaceful conditions restored by Liberation made it possible for the People's Republic to reorganise teaching centres and extensive hospital units in which every recent aspect of modern medicine is considered.

In 1950 the National Congress of Health Technicians made an inquiry into the length of medical studies, which consisted of a short course ($2\frac{1}{2}$ years) and a long course (8 years). It advised four years training for general practice and four years for specialisation (surgery, pediatrics, obstetrics and gynaecology, etc.). At present a new programme has provided since 1959 for much longer courses of six years study.

The students admitted to these courses are very rigorously selected and their instruction is in the hands of members of the Academy of Medical Sciences. An annual quota of the best pupils continue with research in the Academy's laboratories.

Ts'ien Sin-chung has given the figures for Western-trained doctors as follows:

1947	1950	1952	1954	1957
34,600	41,400	51,736	63,046	73,573

The total number of modern Chinese doctors today reaches 120,000, or one for every five or six thousand of the population, whereas fourteen years earlier the norm was one modern doctor for every twenty-five thousand people.

These numbers do not include the 'health officers' or half a million traditional doctors, concentrated chiefly in the southern provinces but also to be found throughout the country. If these are counted, then every thousand of the population has one doctor.

Centres for the teaching of medicine have followed a similar development over the same space of time.

The figures for the university year 1957–8 were: a total of 7,974 teachers of whom 497 were professors, 525 assistant-professors, 2,296 lecturers and 4,656 assistants.

There were then thirty-eight Institutes or Faculties of Medicine plus two of Pharmacy and four of Traditional Medicine. The Faculties of Medicine and Pharmacy had 49,107 students of whom 19,747 were women and 1,909 from national minorities. The women students represented from thirty to forty-five per cent of the total strength, varying according to faculty.

The most important centre is the University of Medical Sciences of Peking. It has grown from 403 students and 134 beds in 1949 to 3,700 students and 2,308 beds in 1965. It comprises Faculties of Medicine, Pharmacy, Stomatology, Hygiene, and Basic Sciences (physics, chemistry and biology).

From 1937 to 1949 it awarded 1,069 Doctorates in Medicine. During the period 1949–65 the number grew to 5,700.

About seventy similar establishments are in existence in the provinces.

The Academy of Medical Sciences, reorganised in 1957, is composed of several sections distributed throughout China: Physiology, Pathology, Histology, Biochemistry, Biophysics and Pharmacy (Synthetic Chemistry and Physiochemistry).

It is the power behind several research institutions devoted to children's diseases, industrial medicine, nutritional defects, epidemiology, haematology and medical biology.

The provinces have not been forgotten. The Hangchow (Che-kiang) laboratory of animal biology was built in 1958. Later came the building of the Institute of Endocrinology and the Institute of Parasitology at Shanghai.

Some half a million doctors, surgeons, dentists, nurses and others have been trained since 1949 to swell the ranks of the public health service which already numbers a million medical workers.

In every large town there are now modern, well-equipped hospitals and each district has one or two hospitals of its own. Every rural community has at least an out-patients' department and the majority of industrial units have their own clinics. The bigger factories and mines also have quite large hospital centres.

Since Liberation the country's institutes of medicine have turned out 120,000 students. In addition some 330,000 young health technicians have completed three or four years of instruction in the two hundred secondary schools of medicine.

Today each province or each autonomous region (with the exception of Tibet) has one or more institutes of medicine including some which allow specialisation. The first institute for the training of specialists in medicine for miners was founded at Tangshan, the centre of the famous coal-mining area of Kailan.

The length of the courses in the institutes varies from five to six years. The doctors are attached to one or more hospitals in which the students complete their instruction. At the present time ninety thousand students are trained in them, eight times the total roll of institutes of medicine in China in 1947, which was a record year for the period before Liberation.

Since 1958 a great emphasis has been laid on the combination of theoretical and practical studies and the equal development of both of these aspects. The students are moreover required to do ten weeks of manual labour either at the university or in urban or rural communities. In this way it is hoped to lay the ghost of the ancient scholar whose enormously long finger-nails proclaimed his scorn for all work done with the hands. The aim is to force the student to graft a second personality on to himself, that of the manual worker he has never been and which he must become. The norm is in fact the manual worker, and the ideal is the manual worker become intellectual. These arrangements are not of course conducive to higher study and research work and they have not been universally welcomed.[3]

Taken as a whole the desire is to train a 'red and expert' staff, or in other words one which is at once politically educated and professionally competent.

The functions of the Ministry of Public Health finally include quasi-official organisations, of which two are especially important. The Chinese Welfare Association was founded in 1938 by Madame Ching-ling Soong, the wife of Dr Sun Yat-sen. It was first known as the Chinese Defence League and was reorganised as the Chinese

Welfare Fund (1945) before it took its present title in 1950. During the war with Japan it conveyed assistance received from all over the world to the Bethune Medical College and the International Peace Hospital, founded by members of the Chinese resistance, behind the Japanese lines. It has since administered maternity hospitals, kindergartens, health centres, etc.

Second of the semi-official organisations, the National Red Cross Society was founded in 1904. It has been a member of the League of Red Cross Societies since 1919. It was reorganised in 1950 and aims to improve health and hygienic conditions through its eight thousand committees distributed in the provinces, districts and municipalities.

In passing we may note the significant part played by Chinese women in accordance with article 96 of the constitution guaranteeing sexual equality. Madame Chu Lien is vice-president of the Academy of Medicine and Principal of the Centre for Experimental Acupuncture. Madame Li To-ts'iuan is the Minister of Health and Madame Sun Yat-sen (Chin-ling Soong) is a vice-chairman of the People's Republic, while more than twelve per cent of the members of the National Assembly are women. There is even a woman general, Madame Li Cheng.

The racial minorities have not been neglected with regard to health arrangements: hospitals, sanatoriums, nursing homes, prophylactic institutions and centres for the prevention of epidemics have been founded for the national minorities in China, and their staffs have increased in proportion to their development. The autonomous region of Inner Mongolia, for example, had few health centres before Liberation in spite of its vast pastoral areas. Today every district (or banner) has its hospital, its epidemic prevention centre, its clinic for mothers and children and its dispensary. There is a health and prophylactic network based on the district hospitals in practically every pastoral area. Sinkiang, Inner Mongolia, Kwangsi, Ningsia and the region of Yenpien all have schools of medicine or a Faculty of Medicine attached to the universities. These establishments always accord priority of entry

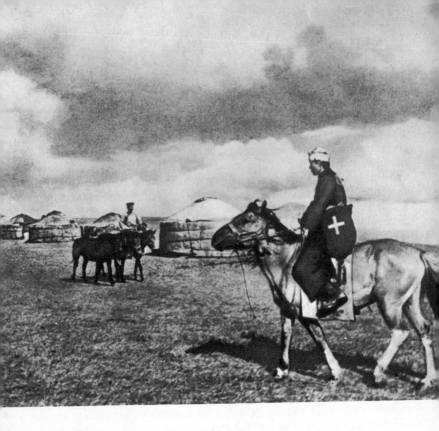

to students from the national minorities. Many such students are also to be found in other schools of medicine: ten per cent of those qualifying at the Peking Faculty of Medicine belonged to the national minorities. Pupils and 'candidates' from the minorities are enrolled in large numbers in the middle-grade schools of medicine and for the medical technicians' courses organised throughout the country.

Epidemics

Cholera was well known to the Ch'ing dynasty. During the first cholera pandemic (1817–23) which began at Jessore, the disease spread to Calcutta and then throughout India. In 1820 it was carried to Zanzibar, and in 1821 it reached Indochina, Siam,

Tongking and China. Wang Hiun-ch'en, the 'corrector of medical errors', described it as a disease characterised by vomiting, diarrhoea and contraction of the tendons (1821).

Epidemics were frequent between 1821 and 1932 and were recorded in the province of Chekiang and in certain areas of Kiangsu, Kwangsi, Kwangtung, Fukien and Shensi. They were particularly bad in Manchuria (1926) and south of the Yangtse (1928). The comparatively low mortality of 1932, which rose however to 7·4 per cent in Shanghai, was attributed to a degree of immunity in the population. Nevertheless the statistics showed more than a hundred thousand victims.

Popular imagery depicted the disease as being characterised by diarrhoea with rice-water stools and vomiting. Numerous cases of cholera were recorded in 1937–9, 1942 and 1946 despite the institution of the National Quarantine Service by Wu Lien-toh, but no further epidemic has been observed in China since 1949. These facts were confirmed by the Health Ministry's Department for Medical Action and the Prevention of Epidemics (1950), and by the work of E. A. Ho, S. M. T'ien (1958) and Ts'ien Sin-chung (1959). They were the result of an ambitious anti-choleraic vaccination campaign. During the pancholera epidemic which was rife in the Philippines in September 1961, the Chinese Red Cross presented more than three hundred thousand doses of anti-choleraic vaccine to the Red Cross of the Philippines.

The plague experienced at Pakhoi (1867) raged through the province of Kwangtung in 1894, and it was during that year that Yersin (1863–1943) made his discovery of the plague bacillus at Canton. In 1944 the epidemic in Yünnan claimed 542 victims, of whom 247 died. Since 1949 the plague has disappeared from Kiangsi. There was another epidemic in masked form in the port of Wenchow (1950), but since then no further case.

Measles epidemics occurred in 1954 in Anhwei and also in 1959–60. Modern treatment by gamma-globulin has been used in combination with a traditional preventive (*Ferula foetida*, *F. scorodosma* B and H; Chinese: *a-wei*) or curative (*Lithospermum officinale*; Chinese: *tzu-ts'ao-chen*).

Japanese encephalitis (encephalitis B) appears to have been described as the summer pestilence in Chang Chung-ching's 'Ailments Attributable to Cold' (*Shang-han lun*). The People's Republic has made a study of its epidemiology and has diminished its virulence by suppressing the mosquito carriers, and by vaccination and antibiotics. Even so, the mortality figure remains between thirty and fifty per cent. Traditional medicine brought an improvement with some thirty antithermics (e.g. *Lonicera japonica* Thunb., *Forsythia suspensa* Vahl.), tonic roots (*Scrophularia ningpoensis* Hemsl., *Rehmannia glutinosa* Libosch, and *R. lutea* Maxim.) and finally nervine sedatives (Siamese rhinoceros-horn and Tibetan antelope-horn, bovine bezoar, musk, tortoise-shell, *Baroos camphor*, *Caumarouna odorata* Aubl.), all of which produced unexpected but interesting results.

Endemic diseases

In response to an undertaking by the Council of State's Planning Committee for Scientific Projects to 'spend three years in a fierce struggle to change the face of the medical sciences', the National Congress of Parasitic Diseases met at Shanghai in November 1958 together with observers and specialists from Russia, Germany, Czechoslovakia, Vietnam and Korea. The vice-chairman of the Health Committee, Ts'ien Sin-chung emphasised the importance of the suppression of the five principal parasitic diseases (schistosomiasis, filariosis, malaria, ankylostomiasis and kala-azar).

Schistosomiasis, an endemic affection caused by a trematode (*Schistosoma japonicum*) contracted in the first place from polluted water, was prevalent on both banks of the Yangtze and in the twelve southern provinces.

In the province of Kiangsu alone 1,255 villages were infested, covering an area of a hundred and fifty square miles (*Chinese Medical Journal*, December 1958). The *oncomelania*, host of the *S. japonicum*, was to be found over a total area of three thousand square miles, and the number of sufferers rose to ten million, forming a threat to the health of a hundred million of the population. This situation was a burden upon the country's economy and was affecting the labour situation. 197 centres for prevention and treatment were set up and split into 1,282 active units employing 17,000 medical technicians. The number of research institutes was increased to forty-two. Initial treatment took the form of a trivalent intravenous injection of antimony potassium tartrate and was followed by a combination of traditional and Western therapeutics. The use of *Veratrum nigrum* was tried experimentally by the 86th Military Hospital. Teams of workers untiringly scoured the most distant country areas and some units treated more than six thousand patients in one month. The results were eloquent: the number of those afflicted, treated in China, was 400,000 in 1956, 500,000 in 1957 and 2,880,000 for the first nine months of 1958. At the end of 1958 schistosomiasis was disappearing completely from more than 167 districts or cities (including the provinces of Kiangsu and Fukien and the city of Shanghai).

Filariosis was rife in fourteen provinces, particularly in the south of Shantung and of Shensi, the east of Yünnan and at Amoy, where Manson discovered the agent of the disease in 1879.

Prophylactic measures have consisted of spraying with DDT and fumigation with BHC (*Chinese Medical Journal*, April 1960). Curative treatment has been by hetrazan, sometimes with acupuncture.

Malaria before the rise of the People's Republic claimed thirty million victims. It prevailed in an endemic state in the southern provinces and in the Yangtze valley, where sixty-six per cent of the population were affected in 1932.

Before 1950 the population of Szemao (Yünnan) fell from forty thousand to a thousand inhabitants. The health service of the People's Republic set up thirty-four centres to combat malaria, staffed by nine hundred specialists and making extensive use of synthetic antimalarial preparations (atabrine, paludrine, neo-paludrine, pyrimethamine, chloroquine, plasmoquine, plasmocide, primaquine) for the treatment of a hundred thousand patients.

The systematic destruction of mosquitos was accompanied by an intensive campaign of sanitary measures. In each district the cleaning of dikes, canals and wells was a national duty, a vast enterprise involving nine hundred thousand miles of drainage and covering an area of more than two hundred square miles of marshland or wells. In the infested regions fumigations and DDT were employed to destroy the vectors, some forty-three species of anopheles. Assistance from traditional medicine came in the form of herbal drugs (*Artemisia apiacea*, the leaves of *Vitex negundo*, and the root of *Dichroa febrifuga* Lour. already indicated by João de Loureiro, 1715–94).

According to Professor Hou Ch'uan-chao there are fifteen known species of Dichroa in India and Malaysia and four Chinese species (*Ch'ang-shan*) with the medicinal variant *D. febrifuga* Lour. In cases of both vivax and falciparum malaria, infusions of *ch'ang-an* produced encouraging results. After two days the fever abated in eighty per cent of the victims, and three to six days after treatment in the last group of patients. The parasites disappeared from the peripheral blood in two to ten days and the only reaction recorded was nausea or vomiting. A hundred cases were also treated by acupuncture (1957), ninety-nine of them vivax and one malariae.

Kala-azar is a leishmaniasis caused by Leishmania-Donovani conveyed by blood-sucking *Flebotomi*. North of the Yangtze river it was endemic in twelve provinces and three autonomous regions. Before 1949 six hundred thousand villages were affected, a third of them in Shantung. In 1950 Professor Wang Shao-tsing, who had studied the disease in Italy, Greece and Israel, was put in charge of the centre for combating kala-azar and was subsequently appointed Director of the Institute of Parasitic Diseases for the province of Shantung.

The classic remedy (tartar emetic) was toxic and of indifferent efficacy. Pentavalent antimonious compounds of foreign origin were more active, but their cost was prohibitive.

An antimonious sodium gluconate prepared by the Hsinhua factory (Shantung) achieved recovery after six days in ninety-two per cent of the cases undergoing the first course of treatment. A second series of injections brought the percentage of those cured to ninety-nine. The manufacture of the drug was raised to an industrial level and promoted by many mobile teams. In this way more than five thousand patients were cured in Shantung, Anhwei and Kiangsu.

But the cure of the remaining four hundred thousand would have taken more than eighty years at this rate, and it was therefore necessary to envisage mass medical action with the participation of the political authorities and the population.

Towards the end of 1958 an army of medical workers twenty-eight thousand strong was in operation against kala-azar in Shantung. The health of tens of thousands was restored, and the achievements in Shantung were repeated elsewhere. More than seven hundred thousand cures were recorded between 1949 and 1964.

Once the medical army was in perfect working order, the time had come to launch an attack on the vector of leishmaniosis (1951). An investigation revealed the existence of thirty species of *Flebotomus*, and the geographical distribution of the dominant species, *F. chinensis*, was shown to coincide with the distribution of kala-azar of which it is the principal carrier.

In order to obtain a better knowledge of *F. chinensis* it was systematically sought out from 1951 to 1954 in the houses, latrines, drains and sewers of twelve villages near Taian. More than thirty-six thousand insects and 2,800 samples of soil rich in larvae were collected. From 1953 onwards similar investigations were carried out in other parts of Shantung, as also in Kiangsu, Anhwei, Honan, Hopei, Shensi and Kansu.

It was observed that *F. chinensis* appears during the latter half of May, reaches its full growth in mid-June and gradually disappears in July and August. As a rule there is only one generation hatched each year. During the day the *Flebotomi* burrow into dark, unventilated corners, holes and crevices. They come out at dusk, and although their flight does not continue for more than thirty metres at a stretch they are active until dawn, sucking the blood of men, cattle, donkeys, pigs, sheep and dogs. They are extremely vulnerable to chemical insecticides and thus easy to destroy. A judicious spraying of DDT or gammexane powder over all the interior walls in the village at the beginning of the season is sufficient to exterminate the insects.

Since 1956 this method has become widespread in Shantung and other endemic regions. The peasants co-operate willingly in the work because they have received first-hand evidence of the extensive results. The insecticides are provided free of charge by the government.

Today it is unusual to see a *Flebotomus* in the Shantung countryside.

In districts affected by kala-azar, dogs can also contract visceral leishmaniosis and become sources of contagion. In order to track down every centre of infection the dogs in the worst affected areas were carefully examined, and every infected animal had to be destroyed as a preventive measure. By the end of 1958 the marrow of 124,000 iliac bones of dogs had been examined. The majority of those in which there was a positive reaction were from Kansu (the north-west) and Liaoning (the north-east), and this factor was related to the distribution of kala-azar in those areas. In eastern China, where kala-azar was most widespread, canine leishmaniosis was on the other hand rare, which showed that the predominance of the disease had no connection with dogs and that the chief sources of infection were of human origin.

Regional differences in the distribution of the disease over the various age groups were also observed. In eastern China the majority of cases were found among adolescents and young adults, whereas in Kansu practically all were small children. These facts revealed the existence of two types of kala-azar. The one current in the east was similar to that met in India, and its victims were young people and adolescents. Few young children were attacked by the disease, and it was rarely met in dogs. In Kansu on the other hand, where canine leishmaniosis was preponderant, the sufferers were more often babies and children, rarely over the age of ten. This was comparable to the situation in the Mediterranean basin and Central Asia. Epidemiological variations of kala-azar in the different regions lead us to think that there are probably two lines of Leishmania-Donovani, but the question needs more thorough research.

The study of wild animals in the north-west and the east of China in an effort to discover the existence of other natural sources of the disease has so far remained negative.[4]

Ankylostomiasis attacked fifty million people, and the number of those affected by the parasitic worm was a hundred million before 1949.

The modern treatment is tetrachloroethylene and 1–bromine – 2 naphthol, the former being slightly more toxic.

The traditional treatment is in three forms: anthelmintic powder (*ch'iu-ch'ung-san*), the so-called yellow treatment pill (*chih-huang-wan*) and a drug called *fei-tzu-wan*.

Ankylostomiasis had practically disappeared from China in 1960.

Social diseases

The benefits of the welfare state are available for workers and employees, who receive free medical attention. Family allowances do not exist in a country where work has always been held in honour and where there is an acute demographic problem which we shall be returning to. There are four hundred million peasants who do not receive national benefits, but who enjoy the medical services of the 74,000 village units which in 1964 were the basic administrative groups.

Tuberculosis was one of the scourges of the China of the past. The number of sanatoria, nursing-homes and spas founded by unions for the purpose of treating pulmonary tuberculosis and chronic illnesses exceeds two hundred, the number of beds provided being over forty thousand. If each bed is successively occupied by six people a year, the total annual capacity for these establishments comes to more than 240,000 patients.

In accordance with present regulations, patients admitted to sanatoria usually undergo a two months' course of treatment which may be extended if it is considered insufficient to effect a cure. During their treatment manual and other workers benefit from all the advantages specified in the rules for industrial insurance: wages paid in full to those who have suffered industrial injury; a 60 to 100 per cent wage paid (according to the number of years of work) to those ill from causes outside their work. In addition, travelling expenses to and from the place of treatment are paid either in their entirety or in great part by the Industrial Insurance Fund. In sanatoria workers are given three meals a day for which they pay half or a third of the cost, the remainder being met by the State. All medical expenses are paid by the administration of factories, mines and industrial undertakings.

The Asiatic and African Students' Sanatorium, founded in 1954, on the southern slopes of the Western Hills (Peking) occupies an area of twenty-five acres. It is fitted with modern equipment and calls on a wide range of Western and traditional therapeutic methods. These include: hygiene, dietetics, chemotherapy, acupuncture and moxas, collapse therapy (pneumothorac, pneumoperitoneum, etc.), bronchial instillations, atomisers and remedial exercises. By 1962 it had received more than two thousand students.

Cancer

Professor Hu of Peking supervises some thirty-three pathological institutions scattered over the whole of China in which, contrary to previous practice, full autopsies are systematically carried out. Among the malignant tumours primary cancer of the liver comes first, followed by cancer of the lung, then of the stomach and, fourthly, cancer of the digestive tract.

In the field of chorionepithelioma Professor Sung Hung-chung's team (Hsieho Hospital, Peking) has produced some very interesting results from the combination of chemotherapy (6-mercaptopurine) and surgery.

At the eighth International Cancer Congress in 1962 a delegation of nineteen members submitted numerous reports on the biology of cancerous cells, carcinogenesis, the control of cancer, the new drugs in experimental use against tumours, clinical study and the pathology of cancer.

Professional diseases

Professional diseases come within the sphere of the Ministry of Labour, and are surveyed by a Centre for the Protection of Labour containing several departments, one of them technological. This central system is in direct communication with the basic provincial units which, in factories, mines, transport centres, constructional and commercial undertakings, have set up sick-bays and convalescent homes, dependent on the unions in accordance with the regulations for industrial insurance, and numbering several millions over the whole country. In this way manual and other workers suffering from benign diseases can be treated at the appropriate time and quickly recover. They also have at their disposal a number of spas: Siaotangshan (Peking), Tsunhwa (Kwangtung), Hwatsingchih (Shensi), Anning (Yunnan), Chungking, Kweichow, and the hot springs of Tibet (Lhasa, Lake Tzegadan and the River Yangpashan).

Silicosis is a disease which has been given special study. The scourge of miners, stone-cutters, glass-workers, potters and all those working on refractory material, it is caused by the constant inhaling of the silica dust to be found in rock or sand. It produces a fibrous condition of the lung and gradual inability to breathe. An example of its destructive effects is provided by the Hunan tin mine where formerly low tunnels were cut into the rock by hand with no ventilation other than what the workers themselves could provide. Silicosis caused an average of nine deaths a day over the sixty years of the working of the mine before Liberation. The words of a local popular song ran:

> Don't let your son go down the tin mine,
> For once in the pit he will never come out.
> Don't let your daughter marry a stone-cutter:
> He will spit black phlegm and make her a widow.

The government of the People's Republic has tried to prevent silicosis by measures aimed at reducing the density of siliceous dust on the site of operations. Each year large sums of money are devoted to the purchase of equipment for dust control in mines and factories under State or local administration. In 1963 forty million *yüan* were spent for this purpose, and the amount for 1965 will be even higher.

When mechanical boring began to be more widespread in mines, the volume of dust became too great to be dealt with by the small fans and hand sprinklers introduced after 1949. The government gave orders that in those places of work where the silica content of floating dust particles was greater than ten per cent it was to be reduced to two milligrammes per cubic metre of air. When siliceous dust is kept below this level there is no possibility of silicosis. Siliceous dust is now controlled in the majority of mines thanks to the combination of better ventilation, flushing and irrigation.

Large ventilators and humidity suppliers are used in the galleries, and their operators must wear masks made of several thicknesses of cloth. After an explosion, centrifugal fans rapidly evacuate dust and smoke. At the entrance to every main gallery a screen of water, which stops automatically when approached, 'washes' the air passing through it. The walls are frequently sluiced with jets of water in order to eliminate any adhering dust. The result at the Hunan mine is that the density of siliceous dust, formerly 200–1,000 milligrammes per cubic metre of air, has been brought below the permissible two milligrammes. Since 1956 not one single case of silicosis has been recorded among the new workmen.

In factories for grinding quartz and glassworks, where there are large amounts of siliceous dust (quartz is 90 per cent silica), the quartz crushers are enclosed, and in addition a double suction plant takes up all the particles. When the material is prepared for the furnace it is kept in a humid condition and the passages it goes through are sprinkled with water to prevent the dust from rising.

In order to ensure the efficient direction of the preventive work, departments for the control of silica have been set up in those provinces where there are a number of industrial undertakings with a preponderance of siliceous dust. Mines and factories have their own special centres to deal with this task, and the miners themselves often invent devices to deal with dust. A miner in the Lungyen iron mine, Hupei province, perfected a small air irrigation tank which completely eliminates the dust in a tunnel six hundred yards long.

The safeguarding of the workers' health is another protective measure against silicosis. Miners working underground are given special attention, especially those who operate pneumatic drills. All miners have two to four weeks holiday with pay annually. Workers exposed to siliceous dust are given free medical examinations, and only last year five hundred thousand of them were given a lung radiography check. If a worker suffers by a disease which might lead to silicosis, such as tuberculosis or a cardiac affection, he is immediately moved to another job where there is no danger of siliceous dust.

The national regulations provide for the transfer to lighter work with no diminution of salary of anyone suspected to be suffering from silicosis however slight the symptoms. Workers who contracted silicosis in the past receive free medical attention either in their own homes or in specialist sanatoria. Those who are no longer able to work may retire on ninety to a hundred per cent of their normal pay.[5]

Surgery

The 8th National Surgery Congress in 1963 showed modern major surgery fully established in China.

Surgeons are successful in making and perfecting – with their own hands and with the help of technicians – extremely complicated apparatus such as artificial kidneys, cardiac pumps, delicate prostheses for limb amputations, artificial hands, etc. This is no small achievement when we remember that the Chinese are far from having all the resources at the disposal of their Western colleagues. Yet the first case of a completely severed hand being successfully sutured was the work of Peking surgeons in 1963.

The number of surgical centres has been considerably increased, so that a patient can be rapidly hospitalised. In the province of Shantung, for example, there was only one death recorded out of 160 cases of intestinal occlusion in 1963. When the patient cannot be moved the surgeon goes to him. Traumatic, reparatory and orthopaedic surgery has transformed the consequences of industrial accidents, thanks to equipment and re-education. Surgery of the liver is on the track of extensive hepatectomy, the result of anatomical and technical surveys independent of comparable Western projects. Open-heart surgery is fully developed, thanks to an apparatus built on the spot (Fuwai Hospital), and the Institute of Cardio-vascular Pathology (Peking) is a model of its type. Urinary surgery makes extensive use of intestinal cystoplasty and ureteroplasty.

The ancient opposition to surgery has now been definitely overcome. The period 1955–65 saw many publications by Western-trained doctors. Recent works include *Surgery* by Shen Cho-fei, the *Manual of Clinical Surgery* by Wu Ying-chai and others, and *Surgical Technique* by Wang Chih-chiun and his colleagues (1957). Fan Chuo-sheng has written on the medico-surgical specialisation of bone pathology and operations (bone grafting, osteotomy, tendon transplantation, arthrodesis, arthroplasty and limb amputation). Professor Huang Chia-sih, President of the Academy of Medicine, produced important works on thoracic surgery in 1965. Wung Wan (Huang Wan) is the author of *Clinical Electro-cardiography* (1957).

The pharmaceutical industry

The traditional pharmacies were run at craftsman level, and the establishment of a pharmaceutical industry of the kind known in the West is a very recent event. Nothing demonstrates this more clearly than the history of the manufacture of antibiotics.

The first attempts to manufacture penicillin in 1946 and 1948 were disastrous, and nothing of value was undertaken before Liberation, but in 1949 the construction of a penicillin factory was entrusted to an excellent microbiologist, Tung Tsun, at present sub-director of the Pharmaceutical Research Institute of Shanghai.

He first took over an old motor-car repair shop while the building of the factory was in progress, and as he was unable to obtain any new equipment he made his own fermenting apparatus by scouring out old tanks and adding the necessary requisites to them. A numbers of workers were engaged, and the first antibiotic factory in China, Shanghai Pharmaceutical Factory No. 3, was officially opened at the beginning of 1951.

The first problem to arise was that of contamination during the fermentation process. Some dozens of batches were wasted in the attempt to produce pure cultures, eliminating the chances of contamination in the spore chamber and improving the fermentation equipment. After six months there was a considerable decrease in wastage.

Two further obstacles arose however: when the solvent had been

178

added, the fermentation filtrate changed to an emulsion and prevented crystallisation and the formation of pure penicillin. Furthermore, the presence of impurities made it necessary to submit the penicillin to repeated concentration and purification, and no technical data were obtainable from abroad, where the manufacturing process was a closely guarded secret. These problems were solved in 1953 and the factory began industrial production.

Several more antibiotic factories have been built in the north, the north-east and the south-west, as also in the more distant regions of the national minorities. Most of their equipment, such as fermentation tanks, measuring instruments, air compressors, ultra-centrifuges and titration and conditioning apparatus, is of Chinese design and production. No foreign equipment has been used in the factories built over the last few years.

The growing production of antibiotics demanded increasing quantities of lactose for fermentation, but this was expensive and brought with it the risk of cutting short the supplies to consumers of milk and other dairy products. In 1958 Professor Chang Wei-shen of the Peking Biological Research Laboratory suggested the use of cornflour, which was cheap and plentiful. The first experiments produced a very poor penicillin yield, but this was successfully increased. The experiments with cornflour have led to the successful use of molasses and glucose, which China produces in large quantities.

Once penicillin was produced, different kinds of antibiotics followed. China now manufactures considerable quantities of the varieties in current use: syntomycin, streptomycin, aureomycin, chloromycin, terramycin, and tetracycline.

Pharmaceutical Factory No. 3 at Shanghai has also succeeded in producing some of the most recent forms of penicillin. In 1960 a new type appeared abroad and was shown to be effective against *Staphylococcus aureus*. In 1961 China successfully produced neo-penicillin 1, which is now manufactured and widely used in hospitals. She has furthermore contributed to the perfecting of several new varieties of penicillin at present under manufacture.

An antibiotics factory
(photograph from *China Reconstructs*).

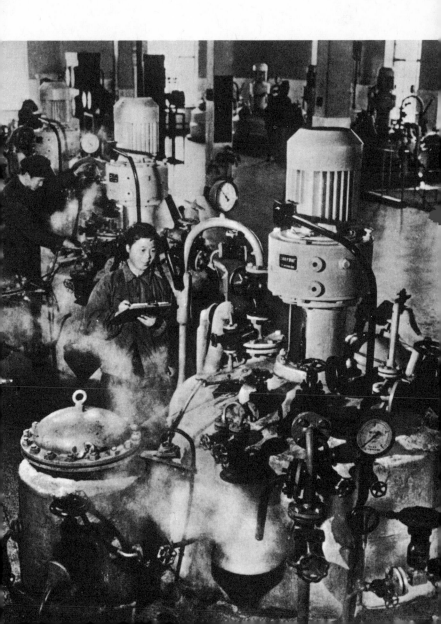

Remarkable successes have been recorded in the field of anti-biotics in China, in spite of the lack of technical data, the initial rudimentary equipment and the poor quality of the reagents. In particular the means have been discovered for making the ion exchange resin used to isolate and purify streptomycin; research continues ceaselessly on the isolation of new sources of antibiotics and on increasing the production capacity of existing sources.

At the second National Antibiotic Congress at Shanghai in the autumn of 1961 some two hundred and sixty reports were delivered. They combined theory and practice and embraced a large number of subjects, in particular the intensified use of antibiotics in medicine, agriculture and stock-raising.

The development of the production of antibiotics has contributed to the promotion of industrial microbiology. Notable achievement has been recorded for example in the fermentation of amino-acids and vitamins, and in the microbial oxidation of steroids. It is foreseeable that industrial biochemistry will become one of the important sciences in the service of the national economy. [6]

When the large factories of Shanghai, Wuhan, Honan and Inner Mongolia went into production, the output for 1962 was sixteen times as big as that for 1957, while 1963 showed a seventeen per cent increase over 1962. About a dozen antibiotics are in current production (penicillin, streptomycin, dihydrostreptomycin, aureo-mycin, tetracycline), and methicillin has now made its appearance.

China has thus made outstanding progress in antibiotic manu-facturing technique. The number of units of potency and the rate of yield show a constant increase, while the consumption of raw materials has on the other hand gone down. So for example at Shanghai in 1962 the number of units of potency for penicillin was double that of 1957, whereas the quantity of raw materials used showed a considerable decrease. The output of units by the North Chinese Factory of Pharmaceutical Products for various anti-biotics has risen to several times its original estimate; its rate of yield in the production of syntomycin has gone up by eighty per cent over the last five years. During 1958 and 1959 the technicians and workers of that factory and of Pharmaceutical Factory No. 3, Shanghai, have succeeded in preparing a new raw material which can serve as a substitute for lactose and bring about a reduction in the cost of manufacture and sale.

In China a penicillin injection today costs about thirty fen, less than a packet of twenty cigarettes. Since 1957 the price has been reduced five times. An extensive range of antibiotics manufactured in China is at present available, and some are exported to other Asiatic countries, to Europe and to Latin America.

The demographic problem

China has lived for long with this problem. Hung Liang-chi (1746–1809), a contemporary of Malthus, showed in 1793 how the population was increasing more quickly than its food supply and how the population might increase fivefold in a hundred years. The forecasts were often confounded by epidemics, floods, emigration, famine and war, but once these scourges had been controlled the situation was again Malthusian.

At present, without counting the overseas Chinese (*Hua-chiao*) and those inhabiting Formosa (T'ai-wan), the population density can be as much as 2,590 to the square mile, and it averages 777 to the square mile in central China. In certain regions of Inner Mongolia, Tibet and Tsinghai the population falls to between two to thirteen per square mile. The average figure is taken as 132 per square mile. The Chinese population density according to Jen Yu-ti (1965) is about 176 to the square mile.

If the six per cent racial minorities are discounted, the Chinese or 'Han' population forms the overwhelming majority (ninety-four per cent). It has reached seven hundred million and is increasing at the rate of twelve to seventeen million a year, more than a quarter of the population of France. This is due to a number of factors: the birth rate, the lower rate of infant mortality and the longer expectation of life.

I Shin-yuan, who made a survey of Chinese genealogy from 1365 to 1914, showed the influence of heredity upon longevity.[7] With a net growth rate of two per cent[8] the forecasts would be a thousand million in 1980 and fifteen hundred million in the year 2000. Assuming a pause in the progression, the figure might be brought down to 868 million, but there is a strong risk of the thousand million figure being reached by the end of the century. The growth rate of the population ought therefore to be brought down to the region of one per cent. That is what Japan has done by means of a spectacular braking operation through the widespread practice of abortion, which is carried out by thousands of gynaecologists.

The classic remedies (increase of employment, growth of sources of food production, the creation of new resources by a transformation in the economy) have never produced spectacular results. The lowering of the birth rate by contraception or abortion, well known to readers of the 'bedroom classics', was the subject of serious study in 1956 but brought no satisfactory solution. Since then China has not ceased to try abortion and sterilisation of either sex, under medical supervision with free hospital attention and paid leave. Attention has been given to the Ogino method, various types of contraceptive, contraceptive prostheses and the inhibition of ovulation. Nortestosterone is now manufactured in fairly large quantities and at a reasonably low price, thanks to state support. Everything, even the old Taoist method (digital compression of the bulbo-urethral gland at the moment of ejaculation) has been recommended. After trying these different techniques, experience showed that the essential need was an appreciation by the masses of the serious nature of over-population. The most varied methods have been used to demonstrate the necessity of birth control.

But the chief method of birth control has been a psychological one. A climate of social and political persuasion has been organised in a fashion unprecedented in human history, aiming at the spread of a degree of chastity voluntarily accepted. Reciprocal supervision, the gathering of young people in a manner which leaves little room for private life, a general puritanism, and a minimum of 'sex' in conversation, popular literature and entertainment have for the time being proved effective; but it will be difficult to extend measures affecting nearly a hundred million young Chinese, among whom, sooner or later, the immense tide stemmed for so long will one way or another break through. What is certain is that there is only a weak and precarious barrier between the extensive real progress effected where life is concerned, and the risk of seeing all achievement in that sector swept away by the catastrophic inflation of the younger generation. Here, as elsewhere, authoritative control is the only way of bringing about the acceptance of a respected policy of family planning. Thus, although the legal age for marriage has since 1950 been eighteen for girls and twenty for boys, it has practically speaking now been raised to twenty-six and twenty-eight (G. Guillain).

5 Traditional Medicine in modern China

At the beginning of the twentieth century traditional medicine still held an important place among the masses, but it began to suffer an eclipse in more cultured circles, either through the influence of dogmatic Europeans or through modernist Chinese ashamed of their past.

The Court medical college was at its nadir; all teaching had disappeared and the care of the Imperial family and its retinue comprised the whole activity of the members. Schools in which traditional medicine was taught were closed one by one, their complete closure being envisaged for about 1929. During the period 1911 to 1948 only eight in fact still functioned.

Yet in a country like China it is very difficult to suppress the whole of the past immediately. The efforts of Li Sheng-chi led to the foundation of a School of Pharmacy at Hangchow in 1913. In 1926 the Society for Pharmaceutical Sciences modified its organisation and set up a commission at Shanghai consisting of nine members, with Yei Han-cheng at the head (*Chu Wen-yeh*, 1941). In 1936 Ching Li-pin, the Director of the Peking Institute of Physiology, invented the term *pents'aology* (roughly, the study of old medical treatises). So the modernist movement, however significant, could not incite millions of peasants to abandon a medicine which was in practice the only one they could appeal to, or to suppress an extensive trade in drugs with centuries of reputation. Although traditional medicine was dormant, it nevertheless went on to prove its irrefutable usefulness, as was the case in Japan, Vietnam and Korea.

At Liberation it was noticed that this form of medicine had been of great service during the foreign and civil wars and that, neither feudal nor reactionary, it was above all the medicine of the people. In view of this it was restored to official esteem in 1949.

Since then specialist hospitals have been set up (in Peking, Tientsin, Shanghai, Nanking, Chungking, Wuhan, Sian, Harbin, Kunming, Nanchang, and elsewhere), as also twenty universities of traditional medicine, chairs of the History of Traditional Medicine, a journal, a pharmacological laboratory, an Academy of Medicine, an Experimental Institute of Acupuncture and Moxa, and a Central Research Institute of Traditional Medicine, founded in 1955. This last Institute is in Peking and co-ordinates the activities of five research services: acupuncture, external pathology, internal pathology, traditional remedies and the history of traditional medicine. The department of acupuncture deals with physiology, physics, biological chemistry, microbiology and etiology.

The People's Health Agency (*Jen-min wei-sheng shih*) published from 1953 to 1956 under the auspices of the Ministry of Health 1,501 different types of scientific and medical works with a total circulation of 23,180,000 copies. The majority of these books are works of reference: dictionaries, works on pharmacy, chemistry and hygiene, medical classics in fact. Thus the *Huang-ti nei-ching su-wen* (photolithographed in 204 pages), an edition giving new punctuation as well as necessary corrections. It is based on the wood-engravings of Chu Tsung-to of the Ming period. There are also about forty medical reviews, half of which deal exclusively with traditional medicine. The 'Review of the History of Medicine and Hygiene', edited by Ts'ien Sin-chung, tries to effect a synthesis of ancient and modern theories. The Peking Institute of the History of Medicine (Professor Li T'ao), the Shanghai Museum of the History of Medicine (Professor K.C.Wong) and the Centre of Traditional Medicine in the Tungshan University at Canton (Professor S.S.Wong) have collected considerable documentary information on early Chinese medicine.

Doctors of Western influence (*si-i*) are in the approximate proportion of one to every ten thousand of the population. Traditionalist doctors (*chung-i*) are in much greater number: one to every nine hundred. The latter have considerable clinical experience and they are able to take over all the anti-smallpox vaccination campaigns. Their therapeutics are economical and they are re-garded as being very efficient in rural and industrial medicine. In 1954 the two groups of doctors were fused together in the *Chinese Medical Association*. This brought about a great change in the mentality of some half a million traditional doctors, schooled

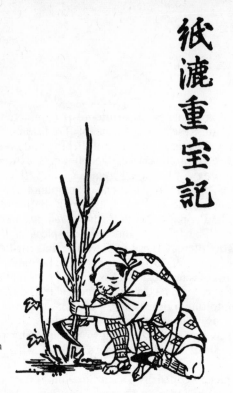

紙漉重宝記

Gathering medical plants in
ancient Japan (*left*) and
in new China (*right*).

after the ancient fashion. No more family recipes or secret processes; no more inferiority complex for a traditional medicine which was neither feudal nor reactionary but, on the contrary, the medicine of the people; no more antagonism between 120,000 modern doctors and the old-fashioned practitioners. Both work together, side by side, in the anti-smallpox vaccination campaigns. In other fields the Westernisers bring to their colleagues their modern procedures of diagnosis and chemical analysis. The traditionalists teach their own great practice and produce results which science sometimes finds difficult to explain. The extraordinary thing is that they have been able to resolve their conflicts and to develop from their buried antagonism a common front against disease, formed from the synthesis of two lines of thought which, though different, are as interdependent as the *yin* and the *yang*. The integration of traditional medicine into Western medicine (the

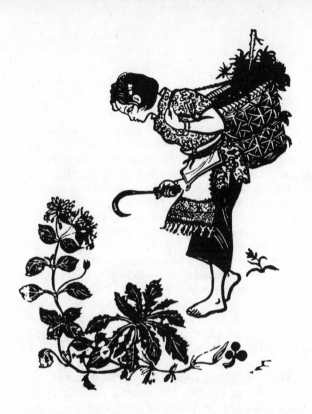

reverse is not possible) is a long and difficult task, but it is of the highest importance for China and for the world, and an achievement greatly to be desired. The theoretical obstacles raised by bringing together doctrines which are chronologically, mentally and scientifically very different are clearly formidable, and the mastery of two such dissimilar forms of thought is no easy matter. Yet the obstacles are not insurmountable, and it is under the combined influence of the east and west winds that acupuncture gives its best results.

We are witnessing in our own time a process similar to the Buddhist invasion of Chinese thought during the period from the fourth to the tenth century. This did not cause the collapse of Chinese thought: by a method of analysis consisting of the interpretation of Buddhism through Taoism (and *vice versa*), Confucianism handled comparative ethics in a way which assimilated it unconsciously into many unacknowledged Buddhist elements, and Buddhism was eventually dissolved in the neo-Confucianism which it had helped to renovate.[1] So traditional medicine and Western medicine have been studied on both a parallel and a complementary basis in China. Western-trained doctors are given further instruction bearing on traditional medicine; traditionalist doctors are introduced to Western medical ideas. Nine-tenths of the staff of a modern hospital are doctors trained on Western lines, the remaining tenth being traditionalist. In a traditionalist hospital the proportions are reversed. The broad plan is first prevention, then integration of the traditional and modern medical systems followed by a similar movement with regard to medical activity in the bulk of the population, and finally the assimilation by world science of everything that is useful in traditional medical knowledge.

The revival of traditional medicine in the People's Republic has not been confined to Chinese medicine in the strict sense. China as a multi-racial country includes dozens of nationalities besides the Han: Mongol, Huei, Tibetan, Uigur, Miao, Yi, Chuang, Puyi, Korean, Manchu, Tungus, Pai etc. The medical heritage of these various racial minorities has not been neglected, and every opportunity has been taken to invite traditionalist doctors to join in the work of the official medical organisation and to hand on their knowledge to the younger generation.

Inner Mongolia's Research Institute for Chinese traditional medicine has a department of Mongolian medicine, as also have certain hospitals. A hospital practising local methods has been founded at Kashgar in Sinkiang. Traditional medicine remains of prime importance in general health organisation and the prevention of disease. Madame Li To-ts'iuan, the Minister of Health (1962), had as her assistants Siun Yun-pei, Chang K'ai, Ts'uei I-t'ien and Chuo Tzu-hua. Classical orthopaedy with its two ancillaries (massage and hydrotherapy) has retained its popular appeal. Tu Chi-ming (*d.* 1961) was its most famous exponent. Li T'ing, a vice-president, was Principal of the Academy of Traditional Medicine (1962), and at Canton Professor Wung Sheng-san (*d.* 1965) was

Dean of the Faculty of Traditional Medicine. Scholars in the field of the history of medicine included Li T'ao (*d.* 1959), Ch'en Pang-hien, Wung Wan and K.C.Wong, Director of the Shanghai Museum of the History of Medicine.

We shall now review the normal course of Chinese medical procedure and follow this with some details on acupuncture, moxibustion, massage, physical culture and traditional pharmacy.

Chinese medical procedure

The timeless, permanent and rather static nature of Chinese medicine has meant that the classical teaching has remained intact.

The *Nei-ching* is still held in honour as a comprehensive work of anatomy and physiology. Traditionalist doctors are indeed convinced that life is the result of a combination in specific proportions of *yang* energy from the sun and *yin* energy from the earth. Human activity, health and sensitivity are nothing other than the refraction of the vital force through the body, which is itself a condensation and materialisation of cosmic energy. After the normal physiology which formed the subject of the *Nei-ching*, Chang Chi tried to categorise man's morbid disturbances into great and small syndromes of which the various diseases are particular examples. This was the substance of the *Shang-han-lun*, a basic work on pathological physiology.

Medical procedure consists of the examination of the patient, the establishment of a prognosis and a diagnosis, and the instituting of a method of treatment.

Clinical examination

Four operations form the basis of the clinical scheme: inspection (*wang*), hearing and smelling (*wen*), questioning (*wen*) and palpation (*tsie*). In pediatrics, called the mute specialisation, questioning is impossible and it is very difficult to take the pulse. Inspection and examination by sound and smell are therefore the only means, and great intelligence and wisdom are required on the doctor's part.

Inspection This is very analytical and leaves out none of the somatic details.

A great deal of information can be obtained from the face, which calls for a meticulous examination of its general aspect, of the forehead, nose, eyes, ears, lips, teeth and mouth, the tongue and its coating, pituitary, salivary and lachrymal secretions. The endosmosis between the microcosm and the macrocosm is effected through the intermediary of the 'openings' and meatuses attached to the sense organs. Each sense organ must therefore be examined both for itself and in respect of the deep-seated viscus with which it is connected.

The nose is the gate of the *ch'i*, and the nostrils are the 'orifices' of the lungs. The colour and temperature of the bridge of the nose, the pulsation of the nostrils and the condition of their mucous membranes are indicative of the condition of the lungs, the spleen and the stomach.

The eye presents a series of peculiar and autonomic changes which are noted in ophthalmological works; but it is also the 'orifice' of the liver and consequently of the other abdominal viscera, in such a way that any affection of those organs may be disclosed by a careful examination of the eye. For this purpose a chart of the eye has been made with the following equivalences: upper eyelid – spleen; lower eyelid – stomach; white of the eye – lung; iris – liver; pupil – kidney; nasal canthus (*nei-chih*) – heart; temporal canthus (*juei-chih*) – heart and small intestine.

The ear also has its own intrinsic symptomatology as well as a borrowed one in its capacity as 'orifice' of the kidney and other viscera. In the ear chart the lobe is shown to be connected with the kidney, the shell of the ear with the spleen and the upper part of the shell with the heart, the tragus with the lung, and the helix ('jade balcony') with the liver.

The tongue is the orifice of the heart, but its chart connects it with other viscera: its left edge corresponds to the liver, its right edge to the lung, its base to the kidney and to the lower burner, its central part to the spleen and stomach, and its tip to the heart. The colour and condition of the lingual mucous membrane, as also the nature of the coating of the tongue have been the subject of a great number of sketches and studies. They are summarised in Yih Hiang-yen's manual of tongue inspection (*Wen-jih-lun*).

The lips, gums and teeth have a less significant symptomatology. The colours noted must first be interpreted in an objective manner, then in connection with the colours arbitrarily attributed to different organs:

Liver blue   *Heart* red   *Lung* white   *Bladder* black

Examination of the limbs is concerned with the nails, the palm of the hand and the sole of the foot. Note is also taken of cutaneous deterioration following eruptive fevers and skin diseases.

Examination of the anus is the rule in cases of fistulas and haemorrhoids. There are several classics which classify the latter into twenty-four varieties.

Uroscopy has not had the success in China that it enjoyed in mediaeval Europe, but the colour of urine, its sediment, volume, and odour are not forgotten. They characterise certain diseases such as chyluria (rice-water urine), jaundice (tea-coloured urine) and diabetes (*siao*) with its three forms (*shang-siao*, *chung-siao*, and *hia-siao*).

Examination of stools includes noting their consistency, odour, colour, frequency, retention, etc.

Auditory perception (quite wrongly called auscultation) affords information on the normal or pathological tone of the patient's voice, aphonia, dysphonia, weeping, laughter, groans, sobs, singing, hiccups, wheezing and coughs. Each of these noises has an organic connection in accordance with the table:

Lungs	*Heart*	*Liver*	*Stomach*	*Bladder*
weeping	laughter	groans	singing	sobs

In bronchitis there are two sorts of cough. The first is the result of an external affection (*wai-chan*) caused by one of six climatic

192

changes (*lu-yin*). It comes suddenly and is accompanied by head-ache, stiffness, shivering and fever. The nose is blocked and the voice is low. There is coryza and dyspnoea. The seat (*pen*) of the affection is in the lung and its effects (*piao*) are in the other organs. It is treated by freeing the cutaneous pores (*ts'ou li*) to allow the heat to escape.

The other kind of cough comes from an internal lesion (*nei-shang*) resulting from one of the seven emotions (*ts'i-ts'ing*) or from excesses in food, sex or work. It appears gradually, the fever is intermittent and the cough is dry with occasional spitting of blood. The patient grows thin and is out of breath. The seat (*pen*) of the disease is in other viscera but its effects (*piao*) are in the lung. It is treated by toning up the *yin* (*pu-shui*) and taking care of the *yang* (pao-yuan) in order to restore full energy to the lung and put the 'Fire of the Void' back into its place.[2]

Questioning is often neglected, since sphygmology affords a diagnosis without the patient's participation.

Palpation of the thorax can lead only to the discovery of tume-factions and superficial vascular pulsations. It has not been de-veloped to any extent.

Palpation of the abdomen, on the other hand, offers a much richer source of information. It can be superficial or deep. It can seek out the points of local, acute pain, or it can bring out points of latent pain by massage. The umbilical region is compared to the bottom of a spirit-glass (*lun-ch'uo*). As the lair of the *shen* (*shen-ch'iue*) and the refuge of the *shen-chi*, 'pivot of the sky and root of life', it is always carefully examined. It affords a means for the palpation of the front of the vertebral column and the lower poles of the kidneys, and for feeling the pulsation of deep-seated blood-vessels. Exploration of the flanks may reveal extravasation, solid, soft, liquid or gaseous tumours and lesions of the liver, stomach, spleen or intestine.

According to the Japanese, seventy to eighty per cent of diseases have an abdominal symptomatology which may take sixteen different forms.[3]

Sphygmology is the essential, and for many doctors the unrivalled method of examination. The complexity of this is best illustrated by the fact that, on one artery, the radial, six different pulses on the right and six on the left may be located, and that there are numerous other arteries to be explored. The classics describe nine whose courses correspond to different meridians: upper orbital, carotid, superficial temporal, radial, ulnar, femoral, deep femoral, posterior tibial and plantar.

There is also the question of the existence of pulses in organs, which was generally accepted at the end of the eighteenth century. There was complete agreement on this point between the West and the Far East, and apparatus was constructed for the measurement of such pulses in France and in Japan.

I. E. H. Niboyet (1951 and 1953) claimed that by pricking a control point on a meridian he was able to bring about chosen modifications in the corresponding pulse. For the study of the different pulses he used a sphygmograph with cutaneous electrodes and thus recorded a deep pulse, corresponding to maximum pressure, a superficial pulse, corresponding to minimum pressure, and a medium pulse, corresponding to a pressure between the other two. A three-track apparatus made an isochronous recording of the three pulses and three pressures. Previously Morita had constructed an apparatus to record the fourteen radial pulses in the form of the pulsogram, in which the graphs vary considerably.

Chamfraut strongly supported the use of indirect piezography (1964). In pediatrics, taking the pulse was almost eliminated from diagnostic procedure and was replaced by palpation of the forehead (for children up to the age of six months) in order to assess its warmth, and by examination of the colour of the pad of the index-finger when massaged from the periphery towards its base (children aged from six months to six years).

According to the *Ling-shu* (1, 13), diagnosis by inspection is lucid (*ming*), by taking the pulse it is intelligent (*shen*), by questioning it is workmanlike (*chung*). To confine oneself to a single method is *chung*, to use two is *shen*, and to rely on the three is *shen* and *ming*.

Diagnosis and prognosis

In Greek medicine, disease, like nature, is intelligible and therefore subject to laws which enable the disease to be identified and its development to be forecast. The concrete thought of the Chinese has driven them in the direction of prognosis rather than towards the diagnosis of disease, diagnosis being the connecting of symptomatology by inductive reasoning to the disturbances which are its cause.

Disease is generally manifested by a symptom which precedes the appearance of other clinical signs. This is the clue which the doctor may follow to his first etiological hypothesis.

The subsequent discovery of an essential feature may enable him to specify the syndrome, a nosological group which often has little in common with our Western norms. Under this general label, and even in the case of monosymptomatic diseases, meticulous examination may bring to light a micro-symptomatology related to individual variations. Many are the systems of classifying symptoms; but no matter how complex, they lie within the framework of the *Pa-chang*, the key to combined diagnosis and prognosis. They make it possible to locate in depth and to define the seriousness and nature of the pathological deterioration in relation to the reactive capacity of the physical system. All the details may be synthesised in an outline of the situation. The *Pa-chang* ('Eight Rubrics' or principles) comprise four pairs of opponents:

yin	*piao* (external)	*han* (cold)	*hiu* (void)
yang	*li* (internal)	*jih* (heat)	*shih* (full)

This is of course a mere sketch of a scheme which we cannot

develop here into all its possibilities, but the majority of diseases fall within this pattern.

Treatment

It may be preventive or curative.

Preventive treatment The curing of the sick but above all the strengthening of the health of the fit is the common thread running through all the classics.

Chinese medicine has always held that if an average doctor is capable of curing a given illness, a great doctor's talent lies in preventing the illness from appearing by controlling it in its latent state.

So Chang Chung-ching wrote, 'Forestalling the ill and treating it before it is apparent is work of a superior order.'

Tao-sheng, *to-tao* and *yang-sheng* are synonymous expressions implying the idea of 'recovering from the outside world elements favourable to life'. This is also the meaning of *wei-sheng* (hygiene).

The Chinese conception of absence of illness rests upon the idea of complete harmony between the body and the world so that when this enosmosis is at its maximum the microcosm may be dissolved in the macrocosm. Starting from the point of sexual and general hygiene, preventive medicine finally arrives in the realms of ethics and mysticism in accordance with the Taoist conceptions. Whatever the case, the parallelism between Heaven, Earth and Man demands a discipline of active behaviour which favours physical culture and the elimination of idleness and over-exertion, a frugal diet, control of emotional and passionate impulses, a degree of sexual continence and a synchronisation of the rhythm of life with the rhythm of the seasons.[4]

Traditional medicine had evolved no instructions from these data with regard to a collective hygiene. But they provided modern China with a basis of mass health education comprising the inculcation of principles of collective hygiene and the prophylactic attack against endemic and epidemic diseases.

Curative treatment The essential principle is for medication to be constantly adapted to each patient's individual case and, in the course of the disease of a single subject, to each phase of its development, taking account of the season, the geographical position and the individual temperament. So, in a very dry autumn, a sore throat with a dry, white-coated tongue indicate humidification with broth of *ts'ing-sao ch'iou-fei*, active in animal glue and *Liriope spicata*. In the Chekiang lowlands the high humidity is a factor to be considered in all external affections; that is why Yu Chen-ch'ou, after giving *su-chiang ta-piao* broth to get rid of the cold of the wind, prescribes *Pachyma cocos*, which absorbs perspiration and avoids the withholding of water. *Sih u* broth is the basic remedy in gynaecology. It is modified according to the patient's temperament. If she is adipose, *Arum* and *Pinellia* may be added to dissolve the humid mucuses. If she is thin, additions of *Rehmannia* and *Pterocarpus* will disperse the Fire. In this way prescriptions are made to suit the individual case.[5] In the words of Chang Chung-ching: 'Individual therapeutics imply not only a special consultation for each patient carried out according to one's own opinion; the treatment and prescriptions will be constantly modified in accordance with the pathological change, if necessary several times in the course of a day.' When, for example, the cure is not making sufficient progress or the illness is not responding, the doctor must know how to keep up an appropriate treatment. But as soon as the disease evolves (unless it is abated) he must adapt his treatment to the new morbid rhythm.

The therapeutist must not be a specialist, but must always concern himself with the whole of the patient's organic and psychological system. He must also pay the greatest attention to the following directions.[5]

1 Respect for the inner breath
2 The use of ambivalent and polyvalent medication
3 The neutralisation of toxins
4 The adjustment of difficulties

1 Respect for the acquired (as opposed to innate) inner breath issuing from the spleen-stomach pairing (*wei-ch'i*) is a condition for the maintenance of life. Since Chang Chung-ching its protection has been a characteristic of medical prescriptions. So, since *shih-tsao* broth contains toxic ingredients like daphne and spurge – acrid, bitter herbs with a harsh action to expel the humours but which may be injurious to the stomach – their violence is mitigated by the predominance of the great jujube which favours the Earth at the expense of Water, thus saving the inner breath. *Lung-tan sie-chan* broth for humid heat and the Fire from the gorging of the ducts of the liver and the gall-bladder, and *ts'ing-wen pai-tu-yin* for high seasonal fevers and heating of the breath and the blood are both acrid and cold; their effect must be mitigated with liquorice which soothes the stomach.

Then again, medical prescriptions make use of drugs which will have a desired action upon each of the *ching* (ducts). Similarly needles or moxas on points located on the *ching* will act either directly on the disease of the *ching* or indirectly on the affection of the viscus which is its source. Knowledge of the *ching-lo* is therefore essential, both for diagnosis and for treatment. Hence the old Sung dictum: to study medicine without the *ching-lo* is to run the risk of error in word and in deed.

2 Frequent use is made of ambivalent and polyvalent medication, sometimes taking into account the whole system in both its deep-seated and superficial parts. *Fang-fung-shen* contains *Siler divaraticum*, sage, mint, *Ephedra*, *Platycodon*, fresh ginger, gardenia, forsythia, *Scutellaria* to purify the heating of the lungs, the stomach and the triple Centre, rhubarb and sodium sulphate to disperse by purging, and steatite to get rid of over-heating by its diuretic effect. This preparation frees externally, purges overheated conditions and facilitates evacuations. It is indicated in external and internal fulness and in fulness of the triple Centre. The action of its many ingredients is not confused but concurrently sudorific, purgative and cleansing. Angelica and white peony harmonise and nourish the blood, *Atractylis* and liquorice harmonise internally and increase the breath. The advantage of the preparation is that it causes sweating without external damage and purging without internal injurious effect.

In other cases the effect desired may be twofold: the support of the 'correct' and the eviction of the 'perverse'. In a system which is perfectly fit, with the 'correct' intact, the rule is first to get rid of all threat of the 'perverse'. But when the system is unfit, or when the 'correct' has suffered from a pathological process, mere eviction of the 'perverse' will not only cause no improvement in the situation but will even prolong and aggravate the disease. The 'correct' must be sustained for action upon the 'perverse' to be effective. There are many prescriptions of this type. *Tsai-tsao-san* and *jen-shen pai-tu san* are at the same time tonic and dispersive. The former sustains the *yang* and causes sweating; it is suitable for cases in which depression of the *yang* is caused by an external affection. The latter acts as a tonic on the breath and frees externally; it is indicated in cases of depression of the breath by an external affection. *Huang-lung t'ang* attacks and has tonic properties. *Chien-p'i wan* and *chih-shu-wan* are resolvent and of tonic effect. All are excellent preparations because they 'walk on two legs'.

Any disease of significance upsets the equilibrium of the *yang* (positive) principle and the *yin* (negative) principle and must be subjected to a treatment which will restore the necessary harmony between this essential pair. If the *yang* principle predominates owing to deficiency of the *yin*, the former (positive) must not be inhibited but rather the latter (negative) must be built up.

Conversely, when there is deficiency of the thermic (positive) principle owing to a predominance of the aqueous (negative) principle, the doctor must take care not to inhibit the latter, but he must build up the former with the classic recipe of eight remedies (*Pa-wei*). Starting from the trigram *Ch'an*, Chang Chung-ching set on either side of a median series of two *yang* (positive) tonic agents of the thermic principle, two lateral series of three tonic agents of the aqueous principle (*yin*, negative), hydratory remedies which eliminate noxious humours.

Thus we have the following formula:

Yin tonics (−)	*Yang* tonics (+)	*Yin* tonics (−)
Paeonia moutan	*Cinnamomum cassia*	*Rehmannia sinensis*
Pachyma cocos		*Dioscroea japonica*
Alisma plantago	*Aconitum Fischeri*	*Cornus officinalis*

It allows a great number of variants, one being the recipe of six remedies (*Lu-wei*). The formula for *lu-wei ti-huang-t'ang* pills is:

25 grammes of the root of *Rehmannia glutinosa*
12·5 grammes of the fruit of *Cornus officinalis*
12·5 grammes of the root of *Dioscorea batatas*
 9·4 grammes of the root of *Paeonia suffruticosa*
 9·4 grammes of the tuber of *Alisma plantago aquatica*, var. *orientale*
 9·4 grammes of the tuber of *Pachyma cocos*

The principal ingredient is *Rehmannia glutinosa*, which, with the remaining five drugs of the prescription, may be arranged as follows:

Tonic	Dispersive
Rehmannia glutinosa	*Alisma plantago aquatica*
Cornus officinalis	*Paeonia suffruticosa*
Dioscorea batatas	*Pachyma cocos*

This formula is in line with the idea that, just as an opening and a closure complement each other, so a tonic effect must be linked with a dispersion. *Lu-wei ti-huang* pills therefore contain three tonics and three dispersives: *shu-ti* has a tonic effect on the kidneys, water-plantain disperses the attendant fire; cornel has a tonic effect on the liver, *tan-p'i* disperses the fire of the liver; *shan-yo* has a tonic effect on the spleen, and *P. cocos* absorbs the spleen's humidity. By dispersing the attendant fire the plantain gives the kidneys the full advantage of the action of the *shu-ti*. *Tan-p'i's* dispersal of the fire of the liver reinforces the tonic action of the cornel. When its humidity is absorbed by the *P. cocos* the spleen responds more easily to the tonic action of the shan-yo. In other words the three dispersives are at the service of the tonics.

So goes the classic argument, but what of Western pharmacology? If the six drugs are given to rats which have been experimentally subjected to a hypertensive nephritis, witnesses report an improvement in the renal function, a drop in arterial tension and a lowering of the mortality rate.[6] Thus divergent explanations lead to the same result.

Other examples show moreover that in the mechanism of drug prescription a tonic effect must be balanced by a dispersal. In *pu chung* broth, ginseng balances orange peel. The tonic becomes fully effective after the perversion has been expelled by the dispersive. According to the *I-fang lun*, *lu-wei ti-huang* pills provide an illustration of this principle. A simple tonic action produces a 'clogging up' of the diaphragm which takes the form of intra-thoracic tension and an aversion from food. The orange peel in *i-chung san* and *jen-shen yang-yung-san*, and *Saussurea* in *chuei-pi-t'ang* prevent this clogging.

3 The neutralisation of toxins is effected by adding an inhibitor to the medication. Aconite administered alone often gives rise to paralysis; this can be avoided by the use of honey, as in the case of the various concoctions of aconite of the *chin-chuei*. *Veratrum nigrum* presents an even more complex situation: a *hemerocallis* of the family *Liliaceae*, its roots are dried, ground, sieved and infused in boiling water. It was known in early times as an effective treatment for abdominal adiposity (*chu*) and modern doctors have used it successfully in cases of schistosomaisis but have noted its toxic effect. An antidote which would not impair the drug's efficacy was therefore required.

It is interesting to see how the problem was resolved in 1959 by a medical team from the provinces of Anhwei and Kiangsu in a symbiosis of Western experiment and traditional opinion.

The poison was administered by a gastric tube to twenty-five healthy dogs for three days, morning and evening on an empty stomach. The minimum lethal dose can thus be fixed at two-tenths of one per cent of the animal's weight. The symptoms of poisoning are first of all nervous disturbances, somnolence and loss of appetite; then, when the full dose has been absorbed, there are the following stages: refusal of food, abdominal distension, arching of the spine, motor disturbance of the hind quarters, slobbering, trembling, dilation and grey discoloration of the pupils, pains which cause the sufferer to cry out when the eyeballs are pressed with the finger, amaurosis, exophthalmia, paralysis of the hind quarters, convulsions, failure to react to heavy pressure on the limbs, dumbness, paralysis, stiffness of the spine and the back legs, occasional delirious yapping; then breathing becomes difficult and the heart-beats, which had accelerated, slow down; their rhythm becomes measured, and at the moment of death breathing ceases before the heart stops beating.

The antidote was discovered by resorting to a classic reasoning. The clinical signs showed a deterioration in the *yin* of the Liver, a lesion in the 'Blood' of the Heart and an exhaustion of the 'Water' of the Kidney. There was deficiency of Water countered by an excess of Fire. When the Water is exhausted, excessive Fire endangers the control of the *yin* of the Liver and unleashes its *yang*. Thus the poison symptoms demonstrate the ruin of the meridian of the Liver with, on the complete consumption of the natural *yin*, the delirious yapping which accompanies death. These ideas led to the choice of bitter-cold, sweet-cold and moistening drugs in order to increase the Water and combat the Fire. By compensating deficiencies and controlling excesses in this way they restore the *yin-yang* balance and suppress the new opposition set up in the system by the *V. nigrum* or the toxic syndrome.

The antidote thus discovered is a mixture of:

1 Two pounds of *Brunella vulgaris* and eight pounds of the root of *Phragmites communis* boiled together with a sufficient quantity of water, strained and reduced to two and a half pints.
2 Four ounces of fresh *Glycyrrhiza*, two ounces of *Coptis chinensis* Franch, three ounces of *pan-lan* and two tenths of an ounce of *Rheum* dried, ground and mixed.

202

3 Pig's bile.

The dose, in proportion to the animal's weight, is ten per cent of
1, eight-tenths of one per cent of 2 and one per cent of 3 mixed
with two-tenths of one per cent of *V. nigrum*.

A new series of experiments showed that this amount taken in
two doses daily for three days was tolerated by the dogs selected.

The principal action is from the *C. chinensis*, more effective in
combination than alone. But the antidote must be administered at
the same time as the *V. nigrum*, for as soon as the poisoning has
reached the stage of pupillary dilation it is irreversible, and the
C. chinensis is inactive.

4 The adjustment of difficulties allows a broadening of the
remedial repertory and the use of agents which would not be easy
to administer alone. It is well known that *C. chinensis*, already
mentioned, is used for dysentery, but it can cause abdominal pains
and vomiting. In *huang-lien-wan* it is combined with *Saussurea* and
Heliocharis which, being acrid and heating, stir up the stases of
Breath and counteract cold bitterness. Thus the bitter element is
reduced, the acrid element rises, and cold and heat are balanced.
There is a direct adjustment and an auxiliary converse action in
order to avoid secondary reactions.

Therapeutics may be purely symptomatic and be applied to what
is immediately visible, i.e. to the branches (*piao*) of the disease. But
the intelligent doctor will strike at the true cause, namely the trunk
(*pen*) which has been hidden by the branches. This he must discover
by using all the resources of the *Pa-chang*.[7]

The eight therapeutic features are: sweating (*han*), expectoration
(*t'u*), evacuation of the bowels (*hia*), heating (*wen*), dispersal
(*ts'ing*), tonic action (*pu*), disintegration (*siao*) and harmonisation
(*ho*).

Therapeutic methods are extremely varied and use a number of
agents simultaneously: *materia medica*, dietetics, physical culture,
psychosomatic techniques, physiotherapy, massage, acupuncture
and moxas. Surgery is resorted to only when all other means fail.

We shall eventually return to the subject of acupuncture and moxas, but it will be profitable first to consider medical therapeutics. Directions on this subject were studied by Sung Chen-sing (in 1958), whom we may follow step by step.

The *Shen nung pen-ts'ao* arranged drugs in the hierarchy of ruler (*chiun*), minister (*ch'en*), deputy or assistant (*tso*) and delegate or servant (*shih*). In the seven recipes (*ts'i-fang*) the *Nei-ching* ordered the ways they are to be associated when prepared according to prescription. The doctor had to learn how to make 'renewed' prescriptions using the association 'master, servant, assistant, envoy'. They were to be centred on a 'master', whereas the associated drugs were to be given in quantities based on conjecture.

Certain drugs have the property of bringing others to the centre of the disease. In the hierarchy they are classified as 'servants' (*shih*). In the *pu-chung-i-chi* infusion for the treatment of a drop in pure *yang* and a deficiency of inner Breath, meadow-rue and hare's-ear 'conduct' the rise of the *yang*. These ingredients are useful in the treatment of both rectal and uterine prolapsus. In *shen-ling pih-shu-san Platycodon* brings all the other drugs to the lung, and there is a tonic effect on the spleen while the lung is protected. In *san miao* pills *Achyranthes bidentata* gives *Atractylis* and *Pterocarpus* the property of reducing and expelling humid heat, so accounting for their remarkable efficacy in cases of atrophy. There are other conductors, too numerous to mention, which increase therapeutic action by bringing the remedy to the centre of the disease.

Each actual case calls for the application of the principles: 'Obedience, Opposition', 'Warm the cold', 'Cool the heated' or some other therapeutic procedure. But if the patient is suffering from debility the need to strengthen him with tonic medication must not be ignored.

There is frequent association of drugs. The great basic prescriptions may contain some hundred drugs, some of which are probably worthless. An example of associated remedies is 'White Tiger' broth, to cleanse an overheated condition and regenerate saliva; it is indicated when a cooling of the *yang-ming* is accompanied by feverish Breath. It consists of:

1 Ruler (gypsum) to eliminate prostration by cleansing the lungs and the stomach.
2 Minister (*Anemarrhena*) bitter and cold, to get rid of the heat and produce saliva.
3 Assistant (non-glutinous rice) to put the Breath of the stomach in order.
4 Servant (liquorice) to protect the Breath of the stomach.

The aim of the combination is on the one hand to reinforce the beneficial action, and on the other to neutralise unfavourable effects. This system is to be found in all prescriptions, but its flexibility makes it adaptable to every situation. So *yue-chiu-wan* has only five ingredients to deal with the six forms of stasis. Cyperus is the Ruler if stasis of the Breath predominates, angelica if it is in the blood, *Atractylis* if it is a mucous or humid stasis, gardenia if it is a stasis of Fire, and yeast if it is in the alimentary canal.

In *lu-wei ti-huang-wan*, *shu-ti* is the Ruler if the blood is low and the *yin* weak, cornel if there is giddiness and a tendency to fainting, *Pachyma cocos* if the quantity of urine is abnormal, water-plantain if there is dysuria, *tan-p'i* if the heart is weakened or overheated by extravasate blood, *shan-yo* if the stomach is weak and the skin dry and rough.

The classic prescriptions can be modified further by additions and subtractions.

The concoction of four ingredients is made of *Rehmannia*, peony, angelica and lovage. But the *Rehmannia* may be cooked or raw, the peony may be white or red, the angelica may come from the top, middle, bottom or the whole of the plant. The effects are different and answer different needs. Raw *Rehmannia* cools the blood; cooked, it will have a tonic effect on it. Red peony activates the blood; white peony nourishes it. The top of the angelica plant works upwards and stops the blood; the middle preserves the inside of the body and feeds the blood; the base works towards the lower part of the body and destroys the blood there; the whole plant harmonises the blood.

The nature of the disease must be clearly distinguished and then the remedies chosen for combining in the prescription. Thus for various blood symptoms the *sih-u* concoction may be prescribed alone: raw *Rehmannia*, the middle part of the angelica plant, white peony and *Conioselinum univittatum* provide tonic effects; the tip of the angelica, red peony and *Conioselinum univittatum* without *Rehmannia* are dispersive.

The concoction of four ingredients, to which *Sophora* and cinnamon may be added, therefore becomes the tonic of pre-eminence. Orange peel may be substituted for angelica, and the addition of *Arum* makes it a 'beneficent recipe'. This is also used with *Aristolochea* and *Amomum*, with *Languas officinarum* and Tamarindus, with daphne and scorpion's tail, with peony, hare's-ear, ginseng etc.

In his 'Ailments caused by the Cold' Chang Chung-ching collected 113 prescriptions following the rule of the 'seven recipes'. Four of these recipes refer to composition and three to treatment.

1 *Ch'i-fang* (odd-numbered recipes). They contain an odd number of ingredients, e.g. one Ruler and two Ministers or two Rulers and three Ministers. These are *yang* prescriptions. Diarrhoea is an 'inner' (*li*) symptom, therefore *yin*; it responds to an 'odd', therefore *yang* prescription, which must however not be used in the case of a sweating patient, for this is a 'surface' (*piao*), therefore *yang* symptom.

2 *Ngou-fang* (even-numbered recipes). They contain an even number of drugs, e.g. two Rulers and four Ministers or two Rulers and six Ministers. They are *yin*. Such preparations will be used to treat 'surface' symptoms such as an absence of perspiration with a fluctuating, hard pulse or a fluctuating, fast pulse. The *yin* treats the *yang* by its opposing action.

3 *Ta-fang* (the great recipes). The disease is polysymptomatic, the disorders acute and numerous. Vigorous action is required for what is called a *yuan* (distant) disease; odd and even prescriptions are used for the treatment, and the 'Great Prescription' will overcome the disease. 'Great' formulas are few in number and consist of powerful drugs in strong doses and converging combinations. For this reason there is the statement 'at least two'.

In this case the *Nei-ching* prescribes 'Deputies' of 'indirect' action in a number related to the number of the symptoms 'in the right direction'.

4 *Siao-fang* (the small recipes). For a monosymptomatic disease in which the disorder of the *ch'i* (breath) is superficial. Weak drugs are given in small doses to deal with the benign symptoms of mild diseases. These 'small prescriptions' have no appreciable effect on the normal breath.

5 *Huan-fang* (slow recipes) of gentle and 'deferred' action, have a tonic effect 'Above' and a remedial effect 'Below'. They have no pronounced defect and are applied to the 'trunk' of the disease. They therefore work by 'modified adjustment' in cases of exhaustion where harsh remedies would be unsuitable.

6 *Chi-fang* (emergency recipes) with both tonic and remedial effect 'Below'. For a case of urgency the prescription must act quickly and it will have a strong flavour. It is directed against ailments which have developed a complication and is applied to 'branch' symptoms for immediate effect.

7 *Ch'ung-fang* (repeated recipes), also called *Fu* meaning 'redoubling'. They are mixed prescriptions in which two opposing drugs are used successively or simultaneously. They are indicated in the treatment of complex syndromes with overlapping symptoms. The work of the Pavlov school may provide some vindication of these opposing combinations.

The prescriptions are directed towards the disease rather than the patient, who in each case will present an individual problem which must be solved in a concrete way by reference to the general clinical situation. Since disease is often caused by deficiency in the vital force, tonics are the medicines most frequently used, whether to enrich and feed the *yin*, to accelerate the breath and the blood, or to strengthen the viscera.[8]

The development of traditional pharmacy has had its economic effects. The production of soft horns on a large scale has necessitated the setting up of centres for the raising of *Cervidae*. Farms specialising in the cultivation of medicinal plants have done away with the need to harvest wild plants in poor economic and sometimes dangerous conditions.

The Chinese pharmacy is extremely well stocked, but we shall confine ourselves to the vegetable kingdom.

The Chinese *materia medica* has made a continuous collection, from the Mediterranean region to Japan and from the equator to Siberia, of all substances which might be used in dietetics and in medicine. Discounting any doubtful products, there are still many therapeutic agents which are of interest for their vitamin or hormone content or for their antibacterial and antibiotic properties. Students of the *pen ts'ao* are continuing their surveys which require the collaboration of the botanist, the chemist, the linguist, the doctor and the exciseman.

Account must be taken of the fact that in a country as extensive as China, regional variations of the same botanical species may have very different names and pharmacological properties. Plants which have been the subject of study during the last ten years include: *Bupleurum falcatum*, a febrifuge; *Coptis teeta*, *Pertulaca oleracea*; *Dichroa* and *Orixa febrifuga*, antimalarial drugs; *Pulsatilla chinensis* and *Brucea javanica*, against dysentery; *Carthamus tinctorius* and *Ligusticum acutilobum*, emmenagogues; *Leonurus sibiricus*, a uterine haemostatic; *Areca catechu*, *Quisqualis indica*, vermifuges; *Corydalis ambigua*, an analgesic; *Aristolochia debilis* and *Eucommia ulmoïdes*, hypotensory drugs; *Coptis japonica*, an antibiotic; *Lagenaria vulgaris* and *Botryopleuron villosulum*, used in ascites, and *Glycyrrhiza uralensis*, active in Addison's disease. In the rhizome of the famous *Panax ginseng*, of the *Araliceae* family, hormones and substances have been discovered which might occasionally be substituted for insulin, cortisone, *Rauwolfia* derivatives and amphetamine, and be free from their side-effects. Further pharmacological surveys will be necessary before we know all the potential properties of this root.[9]

Acupuncture and moxas

The practice of scarification and cutaneous pricking also covers an immense geographical area. It appeared in Central Asia as early as the Neolithic period in the form of stone points (*pien-shih*) and is thought to have reached China from the East.

Acupuncture in its present form is a fully evolved method which is presented to the Western doctor in two different aspects: its incontestable efficacy in certain diseases, and its difficult and disputed incorporation into the present-day scientific medical system.

It is founded on the assumption that to prick the skin will produce a microtraumatism capable of acting at a distance upon a varied range of organs.

In all early medicines ignorant of the nervous system the connections between the different parts of the physical organism were accounted for either by ducts containing blood and the vital forces, or by intangible links (sympathies). Hippocrates recorded the existence of superficial veins in the lower limbs forming a normal connection between the foot and the testicle; cutting them would cause sterility in man. Aulus Gellius (X, 10) reported that Egyptian embalmers had observed a very fine cord going from the fourth finger to the heart, and this idea became widespread in Greece and Rome. Thus the wedding ring was placed on that finger rather than any other because of its connection with the centre of vital heat and of the sentiments. The ceremony of the pledge between bride and groom was therefore founded on a scientific idea.

The Western Middle Ages knew a system of cauterisation and scarification which, by its topography related to the signs of the zodiac and lunations, might suggest a comparison between the zodiacal man of our illuminated manuscripts and the men of bronze or the Chinese charts. In fact no serious analogy has been proved although the idea of links between the various organs did exist.

The Salvatella vein (vein of salvation) was held to link the hand to the liver, the spleen, the kidneys and the lungs. Letting blood from it was therefore considered to have a favourable effect on diseases of those organs. The anatomical interdependence of the uterus and the breasts as an explanation for menstruation, amenorrhoea during pregnancy, and lactation was illustrated by Leonardo da Vinci and accepted until the eighteenth century on the strength of an erroneous angiology.

It can therefore be seen that the idea of working upon superficial structures in order to effect some remote control over deep, inaccessible organs is by no means peculiarly Chinese. It appeared again in a work by Caujolle on the sympathy existing between the cutaneous system and the other systems of the living organism.[10]

But whereas the data remained sporadic and were everywhere left like cupping-glasses, bloodletting and setons to become the stock-in-trade of quacks and barbers, China ordered them into a rational and coherent system which followed a completely individual line of development, though not nearly of the antiquity often claimed for it. It did not in fact become a classic method until the end of the third or the beginning of the second century BC, and for two reasons: the facility of deep insertion presented by steel needles, much less dangerous and painful than their stone predecessors, and the rational vindication of acupuncture through the formulation of a sphygmology and a theory of the circulation of the blood, of the two principles (*yin* and *yang*) and of the vital breath (*ch'i*) closely related to the Indian *prana*, the Greek *pneuma* and the latin *spiritus vitalis*, in a system of ducts (*ching*) some of which have been described only in the Far East. The system was, anatomically speaking, to some extent imaginary, but it must not be forgotten that imaginary anatomy is to be found in all early medical systems deprived of the ability to make extensive autoptical verifications, from Galen until well into the seventeenth century. The original aim of acupuncture was to suppress stasis and restore the normal mobility of the intravascular fluids and *pneuma* either by local bloodletting or by a clearing of the ducts *in situ*. It was also used in order to couch opacity of the crystalline lens, and in this respect the treatment of cataract figures in the great works on acupuncture.

But there developed a quest for indirect action at some distance from the point where the needles were applied, and in some cases the needles were replaced by moxas or even by massage. It cannot, however, be too strongly emphasised that acupuncture was never the only weapon of the Chinese doctor. Dietetics, general and sexual hygiene, moxas, massage, physiotherapy, hydrotherapy, physical culture, breathing techniques and remedies of every order have always been used. Indeed at certain periods acupuncture was neglected as a form of treatment which was either of little effect or dangerous.

As scientific medicine triumphed, based on the concepts of the anatomical fact and the microbe, as the European superiority complex with regard to other civilisations developed, so acupuncture lost its interest and was abandoned by its early champions to be dismissed as quackery and exoticism.

The present revival of interest is due to a progressive reassessment of Far Eastern culture considered in all its elements and to a reaction against that materialist scientific medicine which is preoccupied only with the human machine and not with the sick man as a whole. He has the impression that the acupuncture practitioner gives his problems all the attention and care they need and that he is being made to run no risk. So the patient has complete confidence, a confidence which is justified by the fact that Western practitioners in acupuncture (especially in France) are neither healers nor charlatans, but doctors of medicine who wish to make acupuncture a true specialisation. If it has not yet reached this stage, it is nevertheless the subject of teaching given within the structure of the medical college of the Paris hospitals in the physiotherapy service at the Hôtel-Dieu. Acupuncture consultations are held in the Paris hospitals and municipal dispensaries, at the Institution Nationale des Invalides, at Lyons, Algiers, and elsewhere.

There are about five hundred French acupuncture practitioners. They are members of two French acupuncture societies which are in the process of being combined. Germany, Austria, England, Belgium, Brazil, Switzerland, Italy and Argentina also have vigorous associations under the patronage of the International Acupuncture Society.

While some practitioners of the old school have taken over the obsolete cosmology and adopted an unscientific attitude, others, younger, have been disturbed by the paradox of a method which is indubitably effective in some diseases but (as we have seen) is of difficult and disputable incorporation into the structure of the modern scientific system. They are shocked at using a method which in many aspects is still subjective. Knowing the value of pharmacological experiment, they put their faith in antibiotics, hormones and chemical medicines and hesitate to use such a different and as yet more or less irrational method to treat diseases they can cure in another way.

These hesitations have become fewer since surveys of acupuncture points were carried out with regard to their electrical properties by French, Japanese and Chinese scholars. Niboyet, Pouret, Brunet and Grenier, Yoshio Manaka, Okamoto, Chang Hie-ho and Chu Lung-yu have constructed equipment which, now it is in current use, has transformed acupuncture technique.

These authors have demonstrated the skin's greater permeability to an electric current on the line of the acupuncture points, as opposed to a markedly less permeability to an electric current in the immediately adjacent cutaneous zone. Between two points on the same meridian it is claimed that a zone of less resistance to the passage of an electric current remains perceptible on a body recently dead.[11] The electric current does not pass through this zone in the same way in a pathological case as in a healthy one: in the former the electrical resistance is lowered along the path of the meridian corresponding to the diseased organ. In patients who have already undergone electrical treatment and X-ray therapy all these characteristics disappear.[12] But almost with this sole exception the

Chinese 'points' can be detected by instruments and their electrical resistance measured in micro-ampères. They may therefore be considered to have an indisputable objective existence.

For a long time the effect of acupuncture on a normal individual was misunderstood. It is now known that it acts upon the composition of the blood, the speed of sedimentation, the rates of haemoglobin, fibrinogen, agglutinins and serum haemolysins, the alteration of the Arneth formula, the rate of coagulation, glycaemia, calcaemia, electrophoresis, the reticulo-endothelial system, the endocrine glands, the neuro-vegetative system and the central nervous system. Its effect in the last mentioned case has been recorded by systematic encephalography.

Korean acupuncture specialists have added a radio-isotope to their needle and in this way have traced with a Geiger counter the path of radioactive elements in the human body. There is however much to be done in the study of the physiology of acupuncture with all the resources of modern biological research.

The classic acupuncture techniques have undergone frequent changes. The Japanese differentiated diseases of the *pneuma*, where traditional methods were indicated, from 'diseases of the blood' for which they used thicker needles which would draw a few drops of blood. This minute bloodletting was thought to be beneficial in cases of epistaxis, acute tonsillitis, lumbago and rheumatism, and could be followed by a minute cupping operation. By passing different types of electric current through the needles, electro-puncture (Sarlondière, 1815) and diathermo-puncture (De la Füye) have been produced. It is claimed that the combination of three factors, pricking, intermittent electric current and medicinal ions (ionising acupuncture) has given better results than acupuncture alone, especially in arterial hypertension. Another modification consisted of using a hollow needle instead of a solid one and of making micro-injections of anaesthetic or biological solutions at the Chinese points. In the case of asthma, Manaka and Siegel felt the better for injections of a minute dose of Professor Yaoi's anti-smallpox vaccine at points following the clefts in the lungs and at

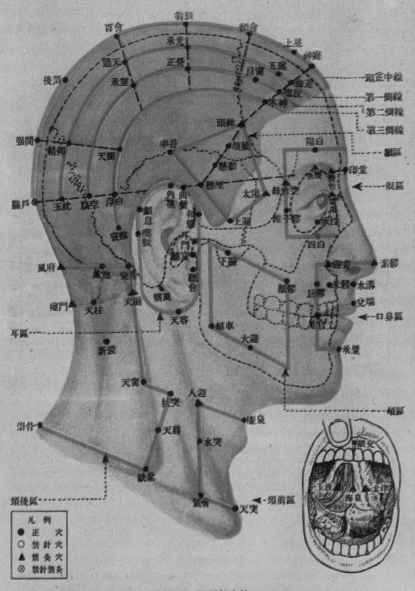

圖一　頭頸部穴位

the sensitive points of the abdomen. Other remedies might be tried, especially in cases where prolonged stimulation of the acupuncture points appears to be indicated.

It has been known since the time of Yang Chi-chou (of the Ming period) that acupuncture, not easily tolerated by children, can be replaced by massage. For further reduction of the traumatism Jean Lamy has invented 'phonophoresis', in which musical modulations take the place of the needle pricks. They are produced by a generator giving controlled frequencies and are transmitted to the skin by means of a vibrator bearing a blunt gold or silver point which is applied to the acupuncture point.

In the majority of cases acupuncture is a mild operation causing little pain. There have however been reports of accidents: discomfort resulting from the use of points of application which were prohibited for reasons of safety or because the patient was suffering from fatigue, and lesions due to deeper effects. It is difficult to draw up a list of diseases curable by acupuncture; one should rather speak simply of patients who have been cured by the method and who are numerous throughout the Chinese world. The diseases concerned include malaria, schistosomiasis, ascariasis, bacillary dysentery, cholera, appendicitis, pulmonary tuberculosis, poliomyelitis, encephalitis B, deaf-mutism, arterial hypertension, enuresis, disturbances in lacteal secretion, tetanus, dysmenorrhoea, rheumatism, neuralgia etc.

But we must remember that in many cases the action of the needles is followed up by all the resources of medical therapy, dietetics and physiotherapy. In contrast to the European tendency, acupuncture is rarely used alone and is not regarded as an all-purpose method.

The field of acupuncture in the West is particularly that of functional disturbances. Essentially it embraces all pains, neuritic: cervico-brachial neuritis, sciatica (except when caused by a slipped disc), lumbago, trigeminal neuralgia, toothache, shingles; or spasmodic: nephritic, hepatic, colitic and ulcerous colics. There has been no report of action upon cancerous pains—nor upon neurological pains except for irregular and impermanent results in paresis, paralysis generally, hemiplegic contractures and aphasia. More notable and encouraging effects have been observed in the treatment of pains in stumps after amputation and disarticulation, and of post-traumatic pains.

It may be accepted that rheumatism (excluding acute articular rheumatism, chronic polyarthritis and rheumatic fever) is in the field of acupuncture. In fact relief has been given to eighty per cent of cases of arthrosis, rather than arthritis, of the arm, leg or spine. The relief may be lasting if the arthrosis is recent, but results are not necessarily related to the radiographic condition of the joint.

In psychiatry the effect of acupuncture is non-existent, and hysterical coxalgic patients have been seen to 'resist the needles but not the electric shock treatment'.

In psychasthenia on the other hand it is equivalent to the effect of tranquillisers in cases of depression, worry, insomnia and nervous disorders, and its action is swift and lasting. But in over-excited patients the effect is not nearly so marked.

Many functional digestive disorders are within the scope of acupuncture. Vomiting in infancy and pregnancy and hiccups will for example respond, as also vesicular disorders. Diarrhoea (but not the infectious types) and constipation, provided there is no trace of a tumour or malformation, are no more difficult to treat by this method than by classical medicine. Allergic diseases such as asthma or eczema give completely inconsistent results: the attack of asthma or eczema may respond in a spectacular fashion, but the illness itself will pursue its course. In the cardio-vascular field, Bouveret's paroxysmal tachycardia, extrasystoles respond well to acupuncture. Similarly in cases of arteritis: if the manometric examinations change little or not at all and the anatamopathology of the arteries is the same, the disturbances may cease and the patient be restored to normal activity. There is no effect in the case of varicose veins.

The use of acupuncture in organic lesions is still very much under dispute.

It has been known for a long time that veterinary surgeons have used it for ulcers of the withers, and doctors for varicose ulcers.

There are now definite examples (quoted by J. Lamy) of the cure of appendicitis, acute tonsillitis, shingles and impetigo of the face, and tick-borne Mediterranean typhus by no other means except a prick made at the requisite time in the appropriate place. The case of appendicitis is worth discussion. With or without the help of medical treatment, acupuncture is able to cure an acute syndrome of the right iliac fossa.[13] Its first effect is the relief of pain. Return to normal is possible if the lesion is in its initial, simply congestive stage. But where there is necrosis or suppuration and fever, the pains and contractures may disappear without the process of perforation having ceased. We know a case in which the acupuncture practitioner had to insist when a surgeon refused to operate on a patient whose symptoms vanished. He could not believe that a simple prick without the association of any drug could be effective to such a degree. He was even more surprised to find a suppurating endo-appendicitis clearly indicative of appendicectomy.

From a simple technique which made a pincushion of the patient's body, as described by Père Huc, acupuncture has become very much more than ingenious needle-therapy. It is of interest to many departments of medical discipline: electro-radiology, physics, physiology, histology, neurology, psychology, psychiatry and internal medicine, not to mention physiotherapy. Like tropical creepers twining from one tree to another in such a way that to pull on one will shake the whole forest, acupuncture has moved in a manner to bring it into all aspects of medicine.

No one therefore may boast that he has mastered all the knowledge at present necessary for a specialist in acupuncture. Yet even though he may, prudently, refuse to treat organic ailments (except at the request of an internal specialist or a qualified surgeon), he must have a thorough knowledge of pain, nervous physiopathology, medical psychology and psychosomatic medicine. Such knowledge will be indispensable to him in order to send on to neurologists and psychiatrists patients to whom he can be of little use alone when he has diagnosed in them a disease of the mind or an authentic nervous lesion.

It would in fact be difficult for the acupuncture practitioner to become a master of his profession if he had not a precise idea of the position of acupuncture both in Sino-Japanese historical medicine and in its continued evolution within present-day medical practice.

Many practitioners would therefore like to see their discipline cease to be a kind of craft in order to become a true medical specialisation practised exclusively by those with examination qualifications. The subjects examined would deal with medical physics, neurology, psychiatry, medical psychology and the history of Chinese and Japanese medicine and civilisation. The examining board, consisting of clinicians, representatives of the basic sciences and an Orientalist, would guarantee the extensive culture required by a modern acupuncture doctor: a knowledgeable doctor aware of the limits of the action of his needles and capable when necessary of appealing to the therapeutic method required.

Acupuncture is encouraged not only in mainland China, but also in Formosa, Hong Kong and the Centres of Traditional Medicine in the Indian Archipelago. Professor Ch'en Tsun-jen, the Director of the Acupuncture Institute, has made an anatomical definition of the acupuncture points with the help of the Department of Anatomy in the University of Hong Kong. He has constructed a life-size copper model which marks the course of the blood-vessels and the pricking points.

In contemporary acupuncture we must distinguish between the didactic school led by Cheng Tan-an and the experimental methods represented by Madame Chu Lien.

Cheng Tan-an (d. 1957), three of whose relatives were famous practitioners, was a pupil of Chiu Chien-chuang and was born in Kiangsu. He set up an acupuncture centre at Wusi in 1930 and after studying in Japan (1932–3) he founded one of the first modern schools of acupuncture and moxibustion at Chengtu. Through his school he provided the new China with a nucleus of acupuncture

A class in acupuncture (*China Reconstructs*).

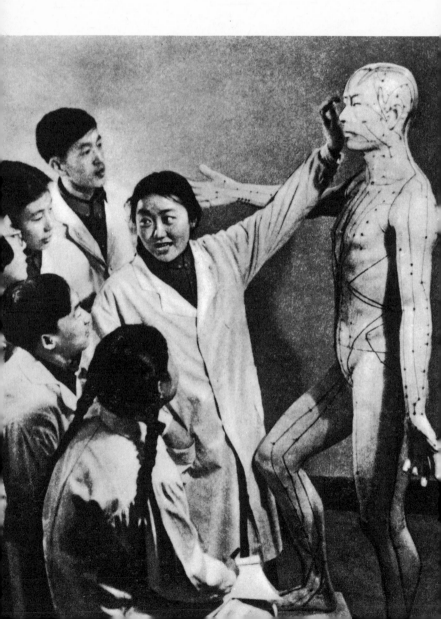

specialists and himself wrote and translated from Japanese authoritative works on acupuncture and moxibustion: a survey of treatments by Chinese needles and moxas (*Chung-chuo chen-chiou chih-liao-hiue*, 1930), commentaries on the survey of Chinese needles and moxas (*Chung-chuo chen-chiou-hiue chiang-i*, 1940), survey of Chinese needles and moxas (*Chung-kuo chen-kiou-hiue*) published by the People's Health Agency (1955, and a posthumous edition, 1959). Cheng Tan-an was also interested in breathing techniques, internal medicine and the study of fevers. He wrote a new commentary on 'Ailments Attributable to the Cold' with an appendix on acupuncture (Kiangsu Health Agency, 1955). He was a member of the Academy of Sciences and vice-president of the Academy of Medicine in 1957.

Madame Chu Lien, vice-president of the Academy of Medicine runs an international centre in Peking to which students of acupuncture have come from all parts of the world. At this centre Siao You-shan, Chang Sie-ho and T'an Shu-t'ien carried out in 1958 their study on the electric permeability of the skin. They regarded an exaggeration of electric permeability as a sign of 'fulness' and a reduction as a sign of 'emptiness'.[14] On each meridian organic deterioration was shown more particularly at certain points which faithfully record the meridian's total condition.[15] These points are in three groups:

1 Those which traditionally correspond to the five elements: *Tsing* (the well) at the tips of the fingers; *Yung* (glory) about the base of the fingers and toes; *Yu* (assent) about the carpus and tarsus; *Ching* (passage) above the wrist and the ankle; *Mo* (meeting) about the elbows and knees.

2 The *Yüan* (source) points which have the double property of tonic and dispersive effects and are sometimes confused with the *Yu* points mentioned above.

3 The *Yu* (assent) points of the meridian of the bladder, forming a line on either side of the vertebral column.

The most generally used are the *Yüan* (Chinese) and the *Tsing* (Japanese). The dermatometer shows the comparison:

1 Two corresponding symmetrical points on the meridian of the same organ, making it possible to detect a loss of balance inside the organ;

2 Two corresponding points on the same side but on different meridians, to detect the predominance of one organ over another.

This type of comparison runs up against the difficulty of irregularities in physiology and assessment. The necessary compensation has been empirically established by Chang and T'an but only for the *Yüan* points.

The electrode may be put in contact with the acupuncture needle when it is in position, but (in our view at least) it remains to be shown that the sign of the intermittent current has the same significance as that of the continuous current used by Siao: negative pole for the treatment of 'emptiness' and positive pole for the treatment of 'fulness'.

Moxas (*chiou*) may have a local or long-distance effect. The pain and the subsequent scarring have restricted their use in the West. The invention of painless electric 'moxators' which leave no trace will perhaps change this state of affairs. Moxa and acupuncture may be combined, either by passing the needle through a moxa already applied or by applying the moxa on withdrawal of the needle.

Moxibustion is indicated in numerous illnesses: various skin diseases, axillo-dorsal anthrax, abdominal swellings stemming from intestinal disorders, precordial pains, anuria, cholera, serious toothaches, insomnia, delirium, nightmares, the resuscitation of drowned and strangled patients, throat infections, epistaxis, dystocia, strangulated hernia, dog and snake bites, rabies, pulmonary tuberculosis, bilharzian splenomegaly, and convulsions.

It is currently used both in hospitals and in Japanese Buddhist temples where bonzes, not doctors (like the ancient Greek priests of Aesculapius), treat large numbers of patients who wish to avail themselves of this popular form of therapy.

Massage

Massage (*ngan-mo*) featured in the *Ling chu* and the *Su-wen* and was held in esteem until as late as the T'ang period. Then (except in the north of the empire) the method fell into neglect and was rediscovered in the southern provinces under the name *t'uei na*. Rules for massage were drawn up by Chou Yu-fan (*T'uei-na yao-kiue*, 1575), Kung Yun-lin (*T'uei-na ts'iuan-shu*), Hia Yu-chu (*You-ch'o chen-ching*) and Wu Shang-sien (1850). The ideograph *ngan* (formerly *na*) is formed from 'hand' and 'rest'. It implies that the hand feels the point to be massaged and stays there, and has the idea sometimes of stopping (*ul ya*), sometimes of pressing back (*kuang-yun*), sometimes of immobilising (*chou ya-fan*).

Light or heavy pressure is exerted with the pad of the thumb, the knuckle of the thumb or two fingers working simultaneously; the palm of the hand is used when dealing with vast surfaces of the thorax and abdomen.

In early times massage was often carried out with the application of unguents. Today an onion and ginger concoction, musk-scented water, or a mixture of the two with spirits may be used. In some cases a small wooden mallet is used instead of the hand.

Massage is carried out by means of a series of different actions:

1 *mo:* vigorous expulsion or gentle dispersal,
2 *ch'ia:* insertion of the finger-nail in place of the acupuncture needle,
3 *jou:* encircling the massage point,
4 *t'uei:* pushing forwards or backwards in a straight line, avoiding the deviations which might bear upon neighbouring meridians,
5 *yun:* to push (the blood) along with a slow, light movement,
6 *ts'uo:* to roll with both hands or two fingers,
7 *yao:* to shake.

The *ch'ia* stops the *ch'i-hiue* (the breath and the blood). It must therefore be followed by a *jou* to restore the circulation by relaxing the *ching-lo* (meridians). The *t'uei* would cause injury if the skin were not moistened. The *ch'ia* is derived from the *ngan*, the *t'uei* from the *mo*, and the *ts'uo*, *yao*, *jou* and *yun* are *t'uei* of the *mo*. *Mo* is a lighter movement than *t'uei* but with more pressure than *yun*. There is a great similarity between these techniques and the Western methods of stroking, friction, pressure, kneading and vibration. The greater number of methods derived from the *mo* than from the *ngan* is due to the more widespread use of the former. We must also add scraping, percussion, trampling and elbow pressures.

Manipulations of the neck, the spine and the limb joints also come within the scope of massage, some types of which may be confused with gymnastics.

The different Chinese massage techniques have been classified by Eric de Winter into three groups:

1 Massage aiming at a local or regional effect is well known in the West. It may lead to a general feeling of well-being or even to a psycho-therapeutic result depending on the relationship established between doctor and patient.

2 Massage aiming to produce results close to or at a distance from precise points of cutaneous stimulation may be called 'reflexogenous'.

   The massage areas may be divided into two groups:

   (a) massage of spontaneously painful points

   (b) massage of selected points, particularly acupuncture points, treated with the hand instead of the needle.

3 Alongside these methods we may consider the Japanese manual resuscitation technique (*kuatsu*) observed by Regnault and E. de Winter. They have shown how reflexogenous stimulation of certain cutaneous zones may produce respiratory and cardiac resuscitation.

Père Amiot, in a letter of 24 September 1790, provided a good example of the first type of massage in his account of the Peking barber-mesmeriser-masseurs. After shaving the scalp they massaged the head, shoulders, neck, spine and tops of the limbs. The movements had their prelude and finale, their *adagio*, *allegro*, *piano*, *forte*, duet and solo. When performed well they had a remarkable restorative effect and produced a general sense of euphoria.

Some masseurs are specialists in the treatment of traumatisms. The combined treatment of limb fractures by traditional and Western methods together saves a great deal of time and leads to excellent functional recovery.

Physical culture

From its earliest times under the Ch'in dynasty (221–207 BC) ancient China loved dancing, physical culture and games, activities restricted with the rise of the Han dynasty, which imposed a literary education on the people and established its triennial competitive examinations in an effort to consolidate the Imperial régime.

In its early form physical culture consisted of *tao-yin* or induction, massage, the mobilisation of the limbs, and breathing exercises. Today *ch'i-chung* and massage are added (*ch'i* therapeutics) together with boxing and sun-bathing.

Hua T'o (AD 136/141–208) was the father of physical culture in the form of the five-animals method (bear, tiger, stag, monkey and crane) discussed on page 224.

As in life, there were two aspects to this method, the one based on immobility (*ch'i-chung*) and the other on movement (*t'ai-chi ch'iua*). They in no way opposed, but complemented each other. The first was regarded essentially as a breathing technique. The breathing action was suspended in order to shut in the breath (*ch'i*), or it was conducted by a concentration of thought (*yin-ch'i*). It was in this way that exhaustion and intermittent fever were treated in the *Nei-ching*. In chronic diseases of the kidney the patient was advised to face south at the *yin* hour, to settle his mind, to retain seven breaths and to swallow the air as if it were a solid substance. The Taoists became interested in the method only after the failure of their alchemy. Under the Eastern Han dynasty they used it for prolonging life and it thus led to the idea of the *tan-t'ien*.[16]

Gymnastics took its name from the *t'ai-chi* symbol, claiming to engender and maintain life by keeping up a healthy movement of the breath and the blood within the body.

Making the animal attitudes his model and as a complement to the well-known breathing methods, Hua T'o invented a form of inductive gymnastics intended to bring man to full attainment of his capacities and reach the normal longevity of a hundred years.

In accordance with the symbol, which is a circle, the movements were circular and the arms and legs were raised to describe countless circles following one upon another.

The trunk and the loins formed 'centres of gravity', the starting points for all the movements which then spread through the whole body.

The limbs were 'like the four wheels of a waggon, the trunk and the loins being the axles'; the motions were continuous like 'the flow of a river', so earning the exercise the name of 'long boxing'. Unlike ordinary boxing, this type, called *fa-siang*, was associated with the work of the breath, *ch'i-chung*, to the extent that breathing and mental training could be an inspiration for physical culture.

The 'method of the five animals' exercised the Essence (*tsing*), the Breath (*ch'i*) and the Spirit (*shen*). But the importance of physical training by concentrating the thought on 'fields of cinnabar' (*t'an-t'ien*) deserves emphasis. Before the gymnastics there had to be a week of *ch'i-chung* exercises, the principle being to set the imagination at rest by banishing all wandering thoughts, what the books called the 'spiritual void' (*hiu-ling*). The main idea was the nurturing of the Breath through exercise, using the individual aptitudes of the animals concerned. One began by deliberately conducting the Breath into the three fields of cinnabar, upper, middle and lower, and one filled them in order to inspire the physical exercise by the fusion of the human body with the animal attitudes. In other words the object was a synthesis transforming 'essence' into 'breath' and 'breath' into 'spirit' and bringing the 'spirit' to its 'void'.

The motions were long and supple, the breathing even, the body relaxed and natural, and it was by control of the will that skilful handling of Fulness and Emptiness was to be achieved. Other preoccupations were to be cast aside and the *ch'i* was to be buried in the 'cinnabar field' i.e. below the navel. Then the 'Full' could be separated from the 'Empty', the *yin* and the *yang* harmonised, the soul relieved, and in a general feeling of ease everything could flow flexibly and the breath could be unified. The basic states were sublimation of the mind, complete control of the muscles and of the chest, flexing of the back, relaxing of the loins, lowering of the shoulders and dropping of the elbows.

The secret lay solely in 'relaxation', presenting a radical difference from the facial contraction, projection of the thorax and abdominal tension characteristic of boxing.

Under the Middle Empire, Buddhism and Taoism encouraged the development of a certain type of physical culture.

With Vedantism, Bodhidharma (Chinese: Ta Mo, *d.c.* 535) brought to China the principles of a physical culture which enabled his monks to relax after a long day of prayer and to defend themselves against secular attack. For this purpose he recommended a series of ten exercises (*i-chin-ching*) for breathing and sensory-motor control in certain desirable attitudes (*asâna*). As abbot of the monastery of Shao-lin in Hunan he perfected a boxing technique in eighteen movements which was given the name *shao-lin*. It became popular among the laity through the influence of the Emperor T'ai-Tsu of the Sung dynasty (960–76), General Yo Fei (1103–41) and the monk Chiao-yuan.

In his Methods for Harmonising the Breathing, Sun Szu-miao of the T'ang period defined *ch'i* therapeutics in six words: *ho, hu, hi, hiu, hi, chuei*.

By the name of 'conduction method' (*tao-yin fa*) the *ch'i-chung* developed extensively under the Sui dynasty with Ch'ao Yuan-fang, and especially also the *wai-chung* or physical culture which provided the five-birds game, the source of the *hing-i, tai-chi* and *pa-tuan-chin* methods of boxing. Boxers then discovered the deep breathing of the Ox (*lao-niou pi-ch'i*) and the conduction of the breath (*yun-hing-*

ch'i), techniques which enabled them to stay awake, to hold back their breathing, to stop their heart beats, and also to receive blows and suffer burns without feeling pain.

After the arrival of Buddhism, five categories of people took an interest in the ch'i-chung: doctors, boxers, Buddhists, Confucians and Taoists.[17]

Towards the middle of the Tang period the *Tao-shih* discovered the original, internal breath, individual to each man (*yüan-ch'i*) and differing from the external breath. In order to conduct the breath (*hing-ch'i*) or retain it (*pi-ch'i*) they invented a type of gymnastics which was not concerned with the external parts of the body. It aimed at an internal effort (*nei-chung*) and involved a more or less constant crouching position.

Deep breathing technique had its influence on boxing, taught in about 960 by Chang San-fung. Contrary to the northern, external form of boxing (*shao-lin* based on muscular strength) *t'ai-chi* was a southern internal form based on suppleness and the art of evasion. The idea was to oblige one's opponent to exert efforts as considerable as they were useless and so put him into an unfavourable position.

Père Amiot gave in 1779 a very precise account of the Taoist *kung-fu* under the Ch'ing dynasty.

A century later Wang Tsu-yuan (1822–97) composed his Illustrated Gymnastics (*Nei-chung t'u-shuo*, 1881) which is a good compilation of all the earlier works. Despite its non-religious character his book was far from being completely secular, and it gave accounts of the Buddhist and Taoist attitudes of meditation (*asana*).

Since Liberation, physical culture has been widely practised in mainland China. The shadow-fight, or *t'ai-chi*, boxing enjoys considerable success and is known in many forms, but the principle is always that of ensuring control of the body through a good breathing training. This technique, suited to the 'honourable age' (sixty, seventy and eighty years) has recently been restored to favour by Tsiang Wei-chiao (1956) and G. I. Krasnoselsky (Moscow

1961). Balneotherapy, heliotherapy, lunotherapy, massage and other forms of physiotherapy may be added to the exercises.

Breathing techniques are also used in therapeutics, when they are called medical gymnastics. The patient is told to eliminate three types of nasal breathing which are pseudo-respiration:

1 *Fung* (wind), a rapid, noisy breathing which drives away tranquillity and scatters the thoughts.
2 *Ch'uan* (panting), an irregular, uneasy breathing which gives rise to phenomena of '*ch'i rebellion*' such as coughing and vomiting etc.
3 *Ch'i* (breath), a strong breathing which, without being noisy, demands an effort leading to fatigue.
4 *Si*, true breathing, fine, condensed and imperceptible. It is maintained by emptying the mind of thought – a condition which it in turn encourages.

This mutual support leads to the acquisition of a state of muscular relaxation and psychical dilution which confers the ability to 'apprehend naturally the emanations of Heaven and Earth'.

Such a state of receptivity is called 'Return to the Roots' and features in all three religions: the Confucians call it *yen-si* (deglutition), the Buddhists *fan-si* (reflex) and the Taoists *chung-si* (sequence).

The twilight condition into which the subject is plunged needs nevertheless a certain vigilance. The first difficulty struck by novices is the unconscious slipping into a somnolence which returns the breathing action to its normal automatic state but at an uncontrolled rhythm which jeopardises psychical stability. This can be avoided by concentrating the gaze on the end of one's nose, which is the origin of the picturesque phrase: 'the eyes like a swinging inn-sign'.

A second difficulty arises from wandering thoughts. One remedy suggested is to count the breaths, but this is not advisable since it makes the simultaneous demand on the attention of supervision of the breathing and mental arithmetic. It is better to reach the required mental concentration with no special means.

Wang Tsung-yo has clearly illustrated the three important points of breathing technique:

1 *T'i sung*, by which, through lack of physical restraint, the thought causes the *ch'i-hiue* to circulate in ducts which have become submissive.

2 *Ch'i-chu*: the *Ch'i* is sent from the chest to the abdomen where it is kept, so as to safeguard the centre of gravity of the body and free the limbs for their mobilisation.

3 *Shen-ning*: uniting of the physical and the psychical, adjustment of the Internal to the External through the six unions:

three external: shoulders with ribs, elbows with knees, hands with feet

three internal: affectivity with intelligence, intelligence with breath, breath with strength.

The expression *Shen-ning* is the equivalent of *yi-shou* in the *Ch'i-chung*, but whereas in the latter neglect of the rule leads to disorders (brain worries, uncontrollable movements, etc.) there is nothing of the kind in the *t'ai-chi-ch'iuan*.

Briefly the method is founded on eight great principles: *yin-yang*, *hiu-shih*, *tsing-t'ung* and *fen-ho*. It is concerned with suppleness and continuity in order to regularise the breath and the blood, just as current medicine is founded on eight principles: *yin-yang*, *hiu-shih* (emptiness – fulness), *piao-li* (external – internal) and *han-jo* (cold – hot).

Breathing exercises are based on immobility, whereas *t'ai-chi* boxing is based on movement.[18] This alternation is in fact a characteristic of life, which for its perfection requires an ascesis to be complemented by another technique.

Yang is born of movement; it is active, positive, sthenic, progressive, hyper. *Yin* is born of repose; it is passive, negative, asthenic, recessive and hypo.

At the present time there are seventy therapeutic units using these methods for the treatment of perhaps a dozen ailments which are difficult to cure; gastric ptosis and ulcers, obstinate cases of constipation, chronic dyspepsia, inactive tuberculosis, neurasthenia, arterial hypertension etc.

In his book *The Practice of the Ch'i-chung*, Liou Kuei-chen put forward the theory that the setting up of new conditional reflexes and 'vestigial reflexes' caused inhibition of the cortex, so exciting the function of subcortical centres and consequently of the Vegetative System. Thus it was claimed that the practice of the *Nei-yang* swiftly changed the blood formula from: Hgb: 15 g. RBC: 4,980,000, WBC: 6,700 (N: 72% L: 27%) to Hgb: 16g. RBC: 5,030,000, WBC: 7,250 (N: 60% L: 32%). The appetite, weight and urine were all increased.[19]

During the course of the exercises, adepts are said to be able by a concentration of the will to produce a principle of longevity in one point of the system, metaphorically called 'the field of the ambrosia harvest'. The hypogastrium or cinnabar field (*Tan-t'ien*) is particularly recommended for men and the epigastrium for women.

6 Conclusion

In concluding a detailed analysis of Chinese medicine it seems reasonable to try to give a general conspectus, setting aside irrelevancies, to bring out both the permanently opposing elements separating the two extremes of Eurasia, and on the other the bridges (as yet very narrow) uniting them.

If we want to understand the doctors of the Far East it will not be enough simply to speak like them (though that would indeed be something); we must also try to reason like them. We must submit to their logic, so different from our own but so satisfactory to them that they regard our syllogistic methods as intolerably heavy and valueless.

Ways of speaking do in fact condition rationalising forms and tendencies: syllogistic in the Indo-European languages, dialectic in the Semitic languages, and parabolic in the agglutinative languages; and the development of a Metaphysics, regarded as a disease of language, has been attributed to a pathological Greek syntax.[1] But whereas the Greek language directed Hellenic thought towards abstraction and analysis, right from the start Chinese pursued the concrete with the tendency towards unlimited singularisation of its monosyllabic word.[2] For want of grammatical categories in which subject, verb and attribute evolve, for want of adequate verbal equipment, Chinese was unable to create abstract and fundamental words favourable to operations of the thought. In such a language Time could be no more than a collection of individual periods, Space nothing but a mass of heterogeneous areas, Jurisprudence a series of concrete cases set the one against the other with no unifying, common doctrine, and the World merely a complex of individual aspects and moving images, excellent for poets but incapable of affording scope for principles of contradiction and causality, the bases of a generalising thought. Although there have been Chinese reasoners and arguers since the earliest times, they have not managed to create a system of logic, but only a concrete dialectic, an art of persuasion, a pseudo-syllogistic method formed outside induction, deduction, analysis and synthesis.

In a medical work the reasoning will often be very brief. The author will hardly have presented one or two arguments before it becomes clear that he already knows how he is going to conclude. This means that in terms of the Aristotelian syllogism he suppresses the major and the minor in order to go on in a few words interspersed with riddles to the conclusion, in accordance with the classic tradition of abridgment, condensation and obscurity. This caused Longobardi to comment as early as 1597 that Chinese reasoning sinned with regard to form (*peccant in materia formae*).

Another point to be noted is that thanks to his confidence in the value of his reasoning, the Westerner is convinced that he has reduced the universe to signs, formulas and laws which will give him one single solution for every problem. The Chinese on the other hand has a pronounced aversion for any deduction carried to its extreme. Every proof which leaves no way out seems to him to be an unreasonable kind of obligation and the mark of an intolerable intellectual arrogance. The principle of contradiction does not appear infallible to him. The idea of cause and effect is far from being of capital significance and he is not put off by the Hegelian principle of the identity of opposites. He has no dislike of ambivalence. To him a thing may be at once itself and something else, itself and its opposite. A problem may allow of several conclusions, neither wrong nor right but simply more ingenious or more profound according to the accuracy of the mind conceiving them. [3] He is therefore ready to accept foreign ideas without any disloyalty to his own values, and to group paradoxical cultural factors in an extremely broad syncretism which, as forecast, does not please the Western mind with its ambivalence, but arouses an antagonistic reaction there. This very individual process of thought relies moreover on a conception of the world which must now occupy our attention, since without it Chinese medical procedure remains incomprehensible.

The Cosmos is a great spatio-temporal conception, graphically represented by the *Tai-chi*. It proceeds rhythmically from an immutable and eternal principle (*tao*) which is manifested either in the form of repose (*yin*), or in the form of movement (*yang*). The succession of the two principles *yin* and *yang* represented by continuous or broken lines makes it possible to form eight trigrams (*pa-kua*). These lead to a symbolic representation of the whole Universe, valid on both a material and a moral plane. It then becomes possible for an ingenious mind to draw from one single trigram the exposition of a physico-chemical phenomenon or historical facts, a topic of military tactics or sexual union, an anatomo-physiological diagram or a therapeutic formula.

The two elements and eight trigrams later acquired the addition of five elements (*wu-hing*) providing means for the explanation of history or biology by supremacy, destruction, or the gyration of the five components of the Universe. There is a conspicuous similarity between the Chinese elements and those of Greece or India in that they all have sequences and oppositions which are justified by a dialectic of antitheses. Two Chinese elements however, Wood and Metal, are unknown in the rest of Eurasia. Moreover the Greek pairs

$$\frac{\text{Cold}}{\text{Heat}}, \quad \frac{\text{Moist}}{\text{Dry}}, \quad \frac{\text{Water}}{\text{Fire}},$$

and especially, in medicine,

$$\frac{\text{Radical moisture}}{\text{Innate heat}}$$

provide better counterparts to the $\frac{\text{Yin}}{\text{Yang}}$ than to other elementary pairings. With this Galenic theory as their starting point the Jesuits could attempt to reconcile Chinese medicine with the Graeco-Latin system which dominated Western medicine as late as the seventeenth and early eighteenth centuries.

The system thus expounded does not fall into line with the Western natural law, derived from the idea of juridical law, which governed this or that category of phenomena independently of the rest of the Universe or of Mankind. Such an idea is contrary to the Far Eastern natural law (*li*) expressing the interdependence of all cosmic elements. Taken as a whole they may be compared to a piece of wicker-work, each element of which is of no interest when considered singly. A single order, valid for all categories of elements and beings, was essential if the harmony of the whole was to be maintained. The Microcosm and the Macrocosm were therefore connected by a complicated system of classifications and values which formed the basis of a system of Aesthetics (by the importance given to the symbol and the allegory) and of Ethics, reflecting the duties assumed by all creatures making up the Cosmos.

In this way a unitary and harmonious conception was formed, closely related to that of the other early Eurasian medical systems. It held that there were elements common to the material world and living beings. The human body was thus a universe in miniature. Conversely, knowledge of the world was by an analogical reasoning a means of knowing man in whom, contrary to the Cartesian dualism, psychology, anatomy and physiology were intermingled and superimposed one upon the other. Disease could be caused by a disharmony between the cosmos and a patient who was unsuited to it, whereupon hygiene would be indistinguishable from ethics. Both quickly stimulated the development of preventive medicine, dietetics, physical culture, gerontology and the study of sex. Such an outlook could not but be favourable to the acceptance of the order of the world as it exists and the importance of leaving it undisturbed. The conception of a 'fate' reserved for everyone, provided it does not lead to inertia, leaves no place for fruitless impatience, stupid agitation and empty rebellion. In its submission to Nature, the Far East practised a kind of duty of improvidence, preferring to leave procreation to the forces of instinct rather than the arithmetic of birth control. It has an extraordinary capacity for endurance, for 'putting up with things', for patience and handing things over to fate, for resisting physical and moral suffering and scorning comfort and material well-being – pleasant things, but in themselves unproductive of those values which are indispensable to the development of a superior, balanced and reasonable civilisation.

And it has been possible to build such a civilisation in spite of the misery and poverty of the rural, rice-growing masses who are imbued with a wisdom which some overdeveloped countries have not yet attained. So psychotherapy holds more importance in popular medicine than tranquillisers and hypnotics. In surgery there have been some remarkable examples of patients' powers of resistance.

What is to be thought as we come to the end of considering the medical system of the Chinese? For reasons already stated, it is based on the coexistence of the Western and traditional systems. Western medicine is now firmly established in a country where the dissolution of the ancient attitudes opens the way for a particularly gifted people to ideas of experimental factuality, scientific knowledge and technical power. Already one Japanese and two Chinese have won the Nobel prize.

Traditional medicine, a faithful reflection of Chinese culture, is a first-rate subject for the human sciences in that it provides an excellent approach to the Chinese and their psycho-affective structure, but it is also not without its interest for Western medicine.

Seen from the comparativist point of view the timeless aspect in which the classic medicine is set is only apparent. It is not because it has kept ancient texts that it has never changed. Its evolution will be the more evident when it has been completely secularised and demythicised, purged in fact of its exuberant cosmology in which some acupuncture practitioners see the very essence of 'their' China.

So, by its dietetic system adapted to a particular environment and climate, by its rich materia medica, by its special techniques (acupuncture, moxas, massage, breathing exercises, substitutes for yoga, hypnosis) it will be able to demand from modern science the reassessment called for. In the excellent words of Professor Jean Filliozat:

> It is important to know the medical systems of Asia not simply as curios of the past but as a store of documentation and knowledge for modern science and medical practice.

Chinese chronology

Shang Dynasty	*c.* sixteenth to eleventh centuries BC	First medical inscriptions engraved on bone or tortoise-shell (*c.* fourteenth–thirteenth centuries BC).
Chou Dynasty	*c.* eleventh century BC to 771 BC	Divination section of the 'Canon of Changes' (*I-ching*), *c.* ninth–eighth centuries BC.
Period of Springs and Autumns	770–475 BC	Pien Ts'io (*c.*430–350 BC ?), founder of sphygmology.
Period of the Contending States	475–221 BC	Fragments of the *Nei-ching* attributed to the legendary emperor Huang Ti.
Ch'in Dynasty	221–206 BC	Shun-yü Yi (*c.* 216–154 BC ?), father of Chinese clinical medicine.
Han Dynasty	206 BC–AD 220	Hua T'o (*c.* 141–207 ?), founder of Chinese surgery. Chang Chung-ching (*c.* 142–212), author of the treatise on 'Ailments caused by Cold' (*Shang-han lun*).
The Three Kingdoms	220–80	Huang-fu Mi (215–82), pioneer in acupuncture and moxibustion.
Western Chin Dynasty	265–316	Wang Shu-ho (*c.* third century), pulse theorist.
Eastern Chin Dynasty	317–420	Cho Hung (281–341), doctor and alchemist.
Northern and Southern Dynasties	420–589	T'ao Hung-ching (452–536), editor of the materia medica of the legendary emperor Shen Nung.
Sui Dynasty	581–618	Ch'ao Yuan-fang, exponent of Chinese etiology (seventh century).

T'ang Dynasty	618–907	Sun Szu-miao (581–682), disseminator of Chinese medical ethics.
The Five Dynasties	907–60	Commentary on the *Nei-ching* by Wang Ping (*c*. 762).
Northern Sung Dynasty	960–1127	Ts'ien I (1035–1117), first Chinese pediatrician. Yang Chiai (1068–1140), disseminator of Chinese anatomy.
Southern Sung Dynasty	1127–1279	Sung Tz'u (1186–1249), pioneer of forensic medicine.
Yüan (Mongol) Dynasty	1279–1368	Liou Wan-su (1120–1200), epidemiologist. Chang Tzu-ho (1156–1260), hygiene specialist.
Ming Dynasty	1368–1644	Li Shih-chen (1518–93), general compendium of Chinese materia medica.
Ch'ing (Manchu) Dynasty	1644–1911	Wang Ts'ing-jen (1768–1831), corrector of medical errors.

We have followed the classical chronology based on the succession of dynasties established by Wan Chuo-ting, completed by Wan Szu-nien and Ch'en Mung-chia (1956), and adopted by a recognised Chinese authority, Madame Feng Yuan-kiun (1958). The reader desiring further details on Chinese matters will find useful the publications of the Institutes of Traditional Medicine (1956–66).

1 Classics

Chang Chung-ching (*c.*200) rev. Ch'eng Wu-chi (1962) *Chu-chiai shang-han lun* (Commentary on 'Ailments attributable to the Cold'). 2nd impression of the 1st edn., Peking, P.H.A.

Ch'ao Yuan-fang *et al.* (610, 4th imp. of the 1st edn. 1958) *Chu-ping yuan-hou-lun* ('Causes and Symptoms of Disease'). Peking, P.H.A.

Chen-chiou chia-i ching ('Classic or ABC of Acupuncture and Moxas') (2nd edn. reprinted 1962, 2nd imp. of the 2nd edn. 1964). Peking, P.H.A. Information kindly supplied by M. Castel of Hong Kong University.

Chen-chiou ta-ch'eng ('Acupuncture and Moxas') (2nd imp. of the 1st ed. 1955). Peking, P.H.A.

Chen-chiou tsi-ch'eng ('Anthology of Acupuncture and Moxas') (3rd imp. of the 1st ed. 1957). Peking, P.H.A.

Cheng Tan-an (1st edn. 1956) *Shang-han lun sin-chu* ('New Commentary on Ailments Attributable to the Cold') rev. Chu Siang-chiun with an appendix on needle and moxa therapeutics. Kiangsu Health Agency.

Huang-ti Nei-ching Su-wen (Simple questions from 'The Classic of Internal Medicine' attributed to the Emperor Huang Ti) (1st modern ed. 1931, 2nd imp. 1955). Shanghai, Commercial Press, 2 vols.

Huang-ti Nei-ching Su-wen pai-hua chiai ('The Classic of Internal Medicine' attributed to the Emperor Huang Ti explained in the spoken language or clear speech) Shantung Institute of Traditional Medicine (1958. 3rd imp. 1963). Information kindly supplied by the Wong brothers.

Li Shou-sien (1798) and Siu T'ien-si (rev. and prefaced 1847) *Chen-chiou i-hiue* ('Simple Study of Needles and Moxas'). After the Sung Classics. Shanghai, n.d.

Pen-ts'ao chang-mu ('General Compendium of Materia Medica') (1959, after the original wood-engravings). Peking, P.H.A. (1956), popular edn. in 6 vols.), Shanghai, Commercial Press.

Pen-ts'ao chang-mu shih-i ('Supplement to the General Compendium of Materia Medica'), 1954, 2nd imp. 1955). 2 vols. Shanghai. Commercial Press.

Shang-han lun shih-i ('Studies on Ailments attributable to the Cold') Research Seminary on Ailments attributable to the cold at the Nanking Institute of Traditional Medicine. Kiangsu Health Agency.

Siu Ta-ch'un (Preface 1759, 1st modern edn. 1956) *Shang-han lun lei-fang* ('Classified Prescriptions from Ailments Attributable to the Cold'). Peking, P.H.A., 60.

Wang Shu-ho (of the Chin period) *Mo-ching* ('The Pulse Classic), new edn. by the Commercial Press, Hong Kong edn. 1961. Information kindly supplied by the Lam brothers.

Mo-ching ('The Pulse Classic') Peking edn. 1962. First new imp. of the 1st edn, Peking, P.H.A.

Wang T'ao (752, 4th imp. of the 1st edn. 1958) *Wai-t'ai pi-yao* ('Medical Secrets of a Civil Servant'). Peking.

Wu Chien *et al.* (1739, 2nd imp. of the 1st edn. 1957) *I-tsung chin-chien* ('The Golden Mirror of Medicine'). Six vols. Peking, P.H.A.

2 Modern works

Chen-chiou-hiue chiang-i ('Commentary on the Survey of Needles and Moxas'). The work of the Shanghai Institute of Traditional Medicine's Centre for Acupuncture and Moxas. 1st edn. 1960.

Ch'en Chiu-lin (Shan Chui-lam) (1960) *Ch'en Chiu-lin lun-i-tsi* (Shan Chui-lam's 'Anthology of Medicine'). Hong Kong, Institute of Present-day Medicine. Information kindly supplied by the author.

Cheng Tan-an (Posthumous edn. 1959) *Chung-chuo chen-chiou-hiue* (Survey of 'Chinese Needles and Moxas'). Peking.

Ch'en Pang-hien (1937, reprinted 1954 and 1955) *Chung-kuo i-hiue shih* ('History of Chinese Medicine'). Shanghai, Commercial Press.

(Shin Hoken) (1940, translated by Narinosuke Yamamoto) *Shina igaku-shi* ('History of Chinese medicine'). Tokyo, Daito Shuppansha.

Ch'en Sin-chien (1963) *Sien-pien yo-wu hiue* ('New Survey of Pharmacology'). 9th edn. Peking, P.H.A.

Ch'en Tsun-jen, with a preface by Professors Shih Chin-mo, Tsin Po-wei, Chang Tzu-chung and Chang Tsan-ch'en (1956) *Shih-wen shang-han-lun shou-tso* (Pocket edition of epidemics from 'Ailments attributable to the Cold'). Shanghai, Health Agency, 75 (1961).

Chen-chiou chih-chu t'u-chien ('Anatomical Location of Acupuncture and Moxa Points'). Presented in the form of anatomy booklets with reference marks to the man of bronze (or copper). Hong Kong, Chinese Acupuncture Institute. Information kindly supplied by the author.

Ch'en Yen-yung (1956) *Wen-ts'iuan ti i-liao tso-yung* ('The Therapeutic Effect of Hot Springs'). Peking, P.H.A. Information kindly supplied by the author (Medical Association of Canton, 1965).

Chu Cho-chen (Coching Chu) and Wan Min-wei (1963) *Wu-hu-hsueh* ('Phenology'). Information kindly supplied by the authors, Chinese Academy of Sciences.

242

Chu Lien (4th imp. 1955) *Sin chen-chiou hiue* ('New Survey of Needles and Moxas'). Peking, 1955.

Chu Lien and Kotcherguine. Professor I.G. (1959) *Rukovodstvo po sovremennoi chen-chiou therapie* ('Manual of Contemporary Chen-chiou Therapy'). Russian version of the above. Moscow.

Chung-chuo chen-chiou liao-fa, also in an English version: 'Chinese Therapeutical Methods of Acupuncture and Moxibustion' (1st edn 1960, 3rd edn. 1964). Peking, Research Institute of Acupuncture and Moxibustion, Academy of Traditional Chinese Medicine.

Chung-i chai-lun (General Theory of Chinese Medicine) (1959). Subjects of study for the Higher Schools of Medicine and Pharmacy presented by the Nanking Institute of Traditional Medicine. Peking, P.H.A.

Chu Yen (1956) *Tsu-chuo chu-tai tsai fu-ch'an-ch'o fang-mien ti ch'eng-tsiou* ('The Evolution of Gynaecology and Obstetrics in Ancient China') *Chinese Review of Gynaecology and Obstetrics*. Peking.

Kuo Mo-jo (1959) *Chung-chuo t'u-nung yo-chih* (Catalogue of the 'Medicinal Plants of China') followed by 220 illustrations in colour. The work of the Chinese Academy of Sciences, presented by Professor Kuo Mo-jo. Peking.

Li T'ao and Pi Hua-to (1956) *Chung-chuo yen-ch'o-hiue shih ta-chang* ('History of Ophthalmology in China') *Chinese Ophthalmological Review*. Peking.

Li T'ao (posthumous article, January 1962) Some early records of nervous and mental diseases in traditional Chinese Medicine, an account in English by Ch'eng Chih-fan and Ch'ang Ch'i-shan *Chinese Medical Journal*.

Li Yen *et al*. (1959) *Chung-chuo chu-tai ch'o-hiue chia* ('Scholars of Ancient China'). Preface by Professor Li Yen. The work of the Peking Academy of Sciences' Institute of the History of Science. 1st edn. Peking, Scientific Press.

Nihon Gakushiin (1955-7) *Meijizen Nihon igakushi* ('History of Japanese Medicine before the Meiji Period'). Nihon gakujutsu shinkokai. 4 vols.

Ogata Tomio (1950) *Rangaku no koro* ('The Dutch School'). Tokyo, Kobunsha. Information kindly supplied by the author.
(1963) *Ogata Koan den* ('Biography of Ogata Koan'). Tokyo, Iwanami shoten. Information kindly supplied by the author.

Ts'ien Sin-chung (1958) *Su-lien pao-chien tsu-chih yu i-shih yen-chiou-so ti ch'o-hiue yen-chieou chung-tso* ('Work and Scientific Research at the Institute of the History of Medicine and Health Organisation in the USSR') Chinese Review of the 'History of Medicine and Health Organisation', Peking.

Tsin Po-wei (1959, 4th imp. 1962) *Chung-i ju-men* ('Introduction to Chinese Medicine'). Peking, P.H.A.

Wong, S.S. (Wong Sheng-san) (1958) *Chi-sing lan-wei-yen yo-wu sin liao-fa* ('New Therapeutic Methods in the Treatment of Appendicitis by Medication') Work of the Centre of Traditional Medicine in the University of Canton supplied by the author. Canton, People's Press Agency.

Wong, K.C. (Wang Chimin) and Fu Wei-Ch'ang (1963) *Chung-chuo i-hiue wai-wen chu-shu shu-mu* ('Catalogue of Publications on Medicine in China in Foreign Languages, 1656–1962'). Shanghai Academy of Chinese Medicine. Information kindly supplied by the author.

(1963) *Chung-wen i-shih lun-wen* ('Catalogue of Articles in Chinese on the History of Medicine'). Lists 6 (1960), 7 (1961) and 8 (1962). Shanghai, Publications of the Museum of the History of Medicine.

Notes on sources

1 The evolution of Chinese Medicine

1 For Maspéro and Bridgman they correspond at least to the penultimate century of the Chou dynasty (i.e. *c.* 320–300 BC), which makes them contemporary with the Greek Hippocratic texts.

2 R. Grousset.

3 Haudricourt and Needham.

4 The date is that given by Bridgman, and not 206 as claimed by C. M. Wilbur.

5 Dated between 167 and 154 BC by Bridgman.

6 The date is according to Fan Hing-chun, one of his most recent editors.

7 Lu Yüan-lei (1956) has collected all the writings on the fever treatise and published them under the title *Shang-han-lun-chin-shih* ('Contemporary Editions of the Treatise on Ailments caused by the Cold'), Peking 1957. From these texts, the Nanking Academy of Medicine's Centre for Research into Illness Attributable to Cold (1959) has produced the *Shang-han-kang-yao* ('Compendium of Ailments caused by Cold'). Another edition has been produced by the Popular Press of Kiangsu province, with notes by Cheng Tan-an and Chu Hsiang-chiun (1956).

The original text of Chang Chung-ching is in the 'literary style' (classical Chinese), not readily understood by the average modern reader. Recent commentaries have therefore reproduced the original text but with a commentary in the national 'spoken language' (*paihua*), which puts it within the scope of everyone. Such a commentary – and even the ancient text itself – is often printed in the 'simplified characters' introduced by the present régime as an aid to universal literacy.

8 Père Roi has given a complete list of the herbal drugs which Bretschneider (1882–96) had first tried to identify botanically in a now outdated work.

9 The last-mentioned edition was published by the People's Health Agency of Peking in 1956.

10 Maspéro.

11 Recent editions have been produced, in 1957 by the People's Health Agency of Peking, and in 1955 by the Commercial Press of Shanghai.

12 Either because of attempts to avoid the inevitable contradictions between the different chapters of the *Nei-ching*, or because a good translation is in fact difficult, we have as yet only partial translations of this great classic into Western languages.

13 In 1956 the Commercial Press of Shanghai brought out the first edition of the *Nan-ching* to copy faithfully the wood-engravings used for the 1368 edition. It contains a complete list of errata, with prefaces, introduction, and an index.

14 This basic work has been translated into Japanese, and it was the most-consulted book of Soulié de Morant, who made a French version of it. The People's Health Agency republished it in 1958.

15 Maspéro.

16 Chou I-liang, 1945. This view has been contested by Needham in his *Science and Civilisation in China*, 1956.

17 We would refer to our own earlier works, to the basic study by R.H. van Gulik (1951), and to the scholarly work of Professors Ch'en Ta-nien and Chu Yen (Peking, 1956).

18 M. Granet.

19 R. Stein.

20 Kaltenmark.

21 Harfeld.

22 Dunstheimer.

2 Chinese Medicine and the Medicine of other Asiatic countries

1 Drs Pham-bach-Cu and Nguyen-van-Huang, representing the North Vietnamese Ministry of Health, made a pilgrimage to the original sources (Peking, 1958).

2 Lee Ki-moon.

3 Doo Jong Kim.

4 A classic which has been reproduced photographically and published in two volumes (Peking, 1957).

5 A photolithographic reproduction with recent corrections by Chinese students of the *pen-ts'ao* has been published by the People's Health Agency (Peking, 1957).

6 Osawa.

7 Hidezurumaru Ishikawa.

8 J. Gernet, 1956.

9 The plants have been detailed by Bernard E. Read (1929).

10 The book has been recently edited by P. Huard and M.D. Grmek (Paris, 1960).

246

11 Renaud and Colin.
12 A partial translation into French of his work has been made by
Dr Nguyên-trân-Huân (1950).
13 Following Albert Sallet (1877–1948), P. Huard and M. Durand have
made an abstract, defining the orientation of traditional Sino-Vietnamese
medicine, of his encyclopedia. In 1942 and 1943, several chapters were
published in Vietnamese Roman characters (*viêt-ngu*) based on the
original Chinese text. Partial French translations have been worked on by
Nguyen-trong-Thât (1923), Nguyên-trân Huân (1951), Truong Tac
Nhan (1952), Nguyên van-Tho (1952), Lê-van-Long (1952),
Luong-Pham-trong (1953), Nguyen-Ngoc-Thang (1952), and
Tran-ngoc-Ninh (1953).
14 Duong-Ba-Banh has given a list of the medical works of this period:
'Introduction to the Study of the Medicine of Viet Nam' (thesis presented
at Hanoi, 1947).
15 Sino-Vietnamese medical techniques have been the subject of works by
Reynaud (1880), Mangin (1887), Mougeot (1894), Le Mar-Hadour
(1895), Estrade (1897), Henry (1898), Baurac (1899), Masse (1902),
Regnault (1900–3), Jeanselme (1906), and Sallet. Medical exchanges
between Vietnam and China are the subject of a comprehensive study by
Professor Feng Han-yung (*Review of Traditional Medicine*, Peking, 1958).
16 E. Balazs.
17 J. J. Matignon, 1900.
18 Blechsteiner.

3 Medicine in China and Europe

1 H. Cordier.
2 Williams.
3 Martin.
4 There were several editions of this fundamental work (in 1680, 1798–1826,
1928), which has also been republished by the People's Health Agency
(1955).
5 Professor Vogralik (Clinical Director at Gorki) published *Chinese
Folk-Medicine* by Ts'ien Sin-chung (Moscow, 1959), giving an extensive
list of popular recipes. I. G. Kotcherguine and Ts'ien Sin-chung produced
Public Health and Medicine in the Chinese People's Republic (Moscow,
1959).

4 Western Medicine in modern China

1 Hughes.
2 W. Grégoir.
3 G. Guillain.
4 Wang Shao-tsung.
5 Ming Chi-chun, 1963.
6 Tung Tsun.
7 In 'Human Biology' 4, pp 46–68, 1923.
8 J. Dresch.

5 Traditional Medicine in modern China

1 Demiéville.
2 Chang Ching-yo, 1958.
3 Nakayama.
4 Yu Chang-cheng, 1960.
5 Wang Shao-hu, 1960.
6 I Ning-yu, Shu Wen and N. K. Koang, 1965.
7 Wang Ch'en-yung, 1959.
8 Sung Chen-sing, 1958.
9 M. Pacquentin: *Histoire et propriétés thérapeutiques du Ginseng* (thesis presented at Montpellier, 1963).
10 Thesis presented at Montpellier, Year X of the First Republic.
11 Niboyet.
12 Brunet.
13 Grégoir.
14 Nakaya and Siao.
15 Nakaya.
16 Li Fang-ts'ing.
17 Yu Ch'ang-cheng.
18 Ch'ao Yung-ts'iuan, 1958.
19 Li Fan-ts'ing, 1958.

6 Conclusion

1 Louis Rougier.
2 M. Granet.
3 Bonneau.

Acknowledgments

Acknowledgment is due to the following for illustrations (the number refers to the page on which the illustration appears): 10, 11, Musée Guimet, Paris; 17, 48, 136–7, Wellcome Museum of Medical History, London; 24, 25, National Library, Rome; 28, 29, 213, Mme Chu Lien; 33, 50, 56–7, 58–9, 63, 75, 79, 96, 99, 105, 149, 218, Authors' collection; 36, 37, 54, 55, 118–9, 120, National Library, Paris; 41, Bibliothèque Saint Geneviève, Paris; 44, 45, Bibliothèque de la Manufacture Nationale de Porcelaine de Sèvres; 67, 68, Variétés Sinologiques, Shanghai; 81, 123, 141, Natural History Museum, Paris; 83, Museum of History of Medicine at the Faculté de Médecine de Paris; 84, 85, 87, Collection of Zensetsu Ohya and E. Hintzsche; 103, École Française d'Extrême-Orient; 107, 108, Medizin in Tibet, Bayer; 111, Professor Rolf Stein; 129, Municipal Museum, Rennes; 156, Professor K. C. Wong, Museum of Medical History, Shanghai; 164, 179, 186–7, *China Reconstructs*.

The map on pages 20–1 was drawn by Mr T. Stalker Miller.

Index

252

World University Library

Some books published or in preparation

Economics and Social Studies

The World Cities
Peter Hall, *London*

The Economics of Underdeveloped Countries
Jagdish Bhagwati, *Delhi*

Development Planning
Jan Tinbergen, *Rotterdam*

Leadership in New Nations
T. B. Bottomore, *Vancouver*

Human Communication
J. L. Aranguren, *Madrid*

Education in the Modern World
John Vaizey, *Oxford*

Soviet Economics
Michael Kaser, *Oxford*

Decisive Forces in World Economics
J. L. Sampedro, *Madrid*

Money
Roger Opie, *Oxford*

The Sociology of Africa
Georges Balandier, *Paris*

Science and Anti-Science
T. R. Gerholm, *Stockholm*

Key Issues in Criminology
Roger Hood, *Durham*

Society and Population
E. A. Wrigley, *Cambridge*

History

The Old Stone Age
François Bordes, *Bordeaux*

The Evolution of Ancient Egypt
Werner Kaiser, *Berlin*

The Emergence of Greek Democracy
W. G. Forrest, *Oxford*

The Roman Empire
J. P. V. D. Balsdon, *Oxford*

Muhammad and the Conquests of Islam
Francesco Gabrieli, *Rome*

The Age of Charlemagne
Jacques Boussard, *Poitiers*

The Crusades
Geo Widengren, *Uppsala*

The Medieval Economy
Georges Duby, *Aix-en-Provence*

The Medieval Italian Republics
D. P. Waley, *London*

The Ottoman Empire
Halil Inalcik, *Ankara*

Humanism in the Renaissance
S. Dresden, *Leyden*

The Rise of Toleration
Henry Kamen, *Edinburgh*

The Left in Europe since 1789
David Caute, *Oxford*

The Rise of the Working Class
Jürgen Kuczynski, *Berlin*

Chinese Communism
Robert North, *Stanford*

Arab Nationalism
Sylvia Haim, *London*

The Culture of Japan
Mifune Okumura, *Kyoto*

The History of Persia
Jean Aubin, *Paris*

Philosophy and Religion

Christianity
W. O. Chadwick, *Cambridge*

Monasticism
David Knowles, *London*

Judaism
J. Soetendorp, *Amsterdam*

The Modern Papacy
K. O. von Aretin, *Göttingen*

Sects
Bryan Wilson, *Oxford*

Language and Literature

A Model of Language
E. M. Uhlenbeck, *Leyden*

French Literature
Raymond Picard, *Paris*

Russian Writers and Society 1825–1904
Ronald Hingley, *Oxford*

Satire
Matthew Hodgart, *Sussex*

The Romantic Century
Robert Baldick, *Oxford*

The Arts

The Language of Modern Art
Ulf Linde, *Stockholm*

Expressionism
John Willett, *London*

Architecture since 1945
Bruno Zevi, *Rome*

Twentieth Century Music
H. H. Stuckenschmidt, *Berlin*

Aesthetic Theories since 1850
J. F. Revel, *Paris*

Art Nouveau
S. Tschudi Madsen, *Oslo*

Academic Painting
Gerald Ackerman, *Stanford*

Palaeolithic Cave Art
P. J. Ucko and A. Rosenfeld, *London*

Primitive Art
Eike Haberland, *Mainz*

Romanesque Art
Carlos Cid Priego, *Madrid*

Psychology and Human Biology

The Molecules of Life
Gisela Nass, *Munich*

The Variety of Man
J. P. Garlick, *London*

Eye and Brain
R. L. Gregory, *Cambridge*

The Ear and the Brain
E. C. Carterette, *U.C.L.A.*

The Biology of Work
O. G. Edholm, *London*

The Psychology of Attention
Anne Treisman, *Oxford*

Psychoses
H. J. Bochnik, *Hamburg*

Psychosomatic Medicine
A. Mitscherlich, *Heidelberg*

Child Development
Phillipe Muller, *Neuchâtel*

Man and Disease
Gernot Rath, *Göttingen*

Mind in the Universe
Gösta Ehrensvärd, *Lund*

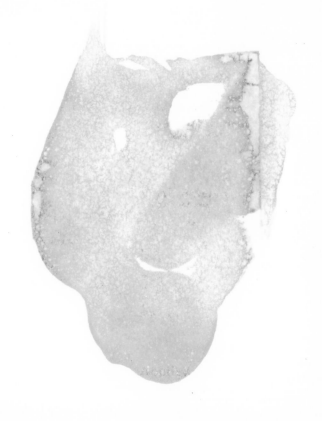